PR

Secrets of the Wedding Night
By Royal Yu (pseudonym)

Category: Weddings/Sexuality
ISBN-13: 978-09787863-5-9
ISBN-10: 0-9787863-5-1
LCCN: 2006909654

Pub Date: 14 February 2008
Price: U.S. $15 – U.K. £10
Pages: 118
Trim Size: 5.5 x 8.5
Binding: Softcover
Illustrated: 21 Illustrations
Backmatter: Chapter references,
bibliography, glossary, index

Rights: Royal Publishing LLC
Distributor: Ingram Book Group

Publisher: Royal Publishing LLC
P.O. Box 2753; Honolulu, HI 96803-2753
Web Site: royalpublishingllc.com

Publicity Contact: Roy Omoto, Managing Agent
Email: romoto@royalpublishingllc.com
Phone: (808) 595-2463

Final Revisions: Text, layout, foreword,
book reviews, back cover, bar code

Secrets of the
WEDDING NIGHT

First Edition

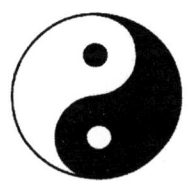

Royal Yu

Royal Publishing, LLC ~ Honolulu, Hawaii
U.S.A.

Secrets of the Wedding Night
By Royal Yu

Published by: Royal Publishing, LLC
P.O. Box 2753
Honolulu, HI 96803-2753
Orders: http://www.royalpublishingllc.com
Author's email: royalyu@royalpublishingllc.com

Copyright © 2007 by Royal Publishing, LLC
ISBN 0-9787863-5-1
First Edition printed in the United States of America

Library of Congress Control Number: 2006909654

Library of Congress Cataloging-in-Publication Data
Yu, Royal
Secrets of the wedding night.
1. Organs of orgasm. 2. Three V's. 3. Three E's.
4. Sex drive. 5. Foreplay. 6. Sexplay. 7. Orgasm.
8. Afterplay. 9. Conclusion.
Includes: Chapter references, bibliography, glossary, and index.

The publisher has made every effort to trace the copyright holders for borrowed material. If any have been inadvertently overlooked, the publisher shall be pleased to make the necessary arrangements at the first opportunity.

Credits: Fig. 1.6 from *Grant's Atlas of Anatomy*, 2005, by permission from Lippincott, Williams & Wilkin.

All other illustrations by Royal Publishing, LLC

TABLE OF CONTENTS ~ Page

DEDICATION

This book is dedicated to my loving wife, four children and their spouses, seven grandchildren, and all of their children's children.

My best wishes to you and yours for a happy and lifelong marriage! My hope is that you may learn and enjoy the secrets about "the birds and the bees."

ACKNOWLEDGMENTS

Many thanks to my copy editors, Lee Motteler and others, who have made me grammatically correct and watched my p's and q's.

WARNING & DISCLOSURES

This book is exclusively for *mature* adults who are married or contemplating marriage. However, if you are offended by explicit descriptions of the human sex act, watch out!

Every effort has been made to provide up-to-date, accurate, and in-depth information on human sexuality, namely the male and female sex acts.

The book is not about kinky, oral, same, or solo sex. It is not about contraception, sexual dysfunction, or sexually transmitted diseases, and does not refer to surveys or statistics.

The text is based on the author's ideas, fantasies, knowledge, opinions, and experiences. The information presented herein is not intended to replace the services of trained health professionals. If mental or physical health assistance is needed, please see a physician.

The names "Jasmine" and "Kevin" are used solely for gender identification and reading interest. Any association to actual persons is purely coincidental.

The author, publisher, and any other entity connected with this book assume no liability or responsibility to any person or entity for any loss or damage that may have been caused directly or indirectly by the information that may or may not have been presented herein. After the author is notified, revisions for any errors or omissions may be considered for incorporation into subsequent editions.

INTRODUCTION

For all the book knowledge that is available today, for all of the new ideals of freedom and emphasis on personal growth, marriage is still about two people, in this example Jasmine and Kevin, who exchange solemn vows to meet each other's needs for a lifetime. They marry for love and they marry for sex, because marriage sanctifies their lovemaking and satisfies their longing for a family.

This is a book for people who are interested in the secrets of how Jasmine and Kevin mysteriously merge into one during the wedding night.

The first half of the book reveals the secrets of anatomy, as the secrets of the organs of orgasm – Jasmine's clitoris and Kevin's penis – are found first. To navigate properly, Kevin might need an orientation of Jasmine's Three V's, especially her vagina. Orgasms are always hard to come by without the secrets of erection, emission, and ejaculation. And it might not be a bad idea for Jasmine and Kevin to learn some of the secrets about their libidos before they begin.

In the second half of the book, they begin with prolonged petting. After only a brief period of sexplay, Jasmine and Kevin are ready to climb to the peaks of their out-of-this-world orgasms. Later, they find out why the success of their marriage could depend heavily on the secrets of addictive afterplay.

When you're ready to find the *Secrets of the Wedding Night,* turn to Chapter 1. But if you're not interested in anatomy or just can't wait, fast forward to the first phase of sex in Chapter 5.

In the 21st Century, images of the sex act are available – everywhere. But there is hardly any reliable information, even on the Internet, about marital sex. Throughout history, not much has been revealed about the sex act, probably because it is the most intimate and secretive activity in a marriage.

Details of what takes place during the wedding night are not found in books about marriage or weddings. And certainly, marital sex (and its secrets) may not be a topic of discussion, especially among married people. Sex in a marriage is just too – taboo!

It doesn't matter whether you do it three times a day, at least 200 times a year, only once in awhile, or even if you've never done it before, it's no secret that sex is also the most complicated activity in a marriage. But there's no need to worry, of course, because no one does it wrong. Still, with the *Secrets of the Wedding Night,* your future martial sex experiences could be absolutely priceless!

chapter

1 Secrets of the Organs of Orgasm

Jasmine's Clitoris and Kevin's Penis

After the perfect wedding reception, Jasmine and Kevin head straight to the honeymoon suite. Before entering, they embrace and express their love with another passionate kiss. Kevin carries Jasmine over the threshold, and they begin their new roles in life as husband and wife as the wedding night unfolds.

Easing Jasmine down on the couch, Kevin takes out a small book titled, *Secrets of the Wedding Night.*

"Just before we left, Jazzy, my father slipped me this book," Kevin begins. *"He told me that he wrote it especially for us, to demystify the myths about marital sex."*

"It was thoughtful of him, but really, Kev, I don't think that we need any advice about that," Jasmine replies. *"Besides, you know how to do it, right?*

"Well, Jazzy, maybe we could take a quick look at some of the secrets," Kevin suggests. *"Perhaps we can learn something new before we start playing."*

"Okay, Kevin, I'm getting curious now," Jasmine answers. *"Hmmm, how many secrets will we find?"*

1

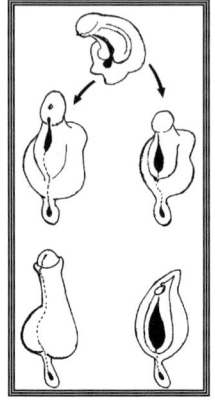

<u>Figure 1.1</u>

Because Jasmine's and Kevin's organs of orgasm originated from the same primitive sex organ, many of their parts are identically named.

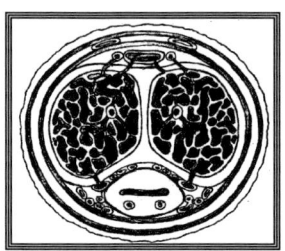

<u>Figure 1.2</u>

For example, the cross-section of the body of Kevin's penis shows three erectile bodies (Fig. 1.2). Each erectile body (corpus cavernosum, penis), of the two larger ones, tapers into a leg (crus, penis) that is connected to the pubis bone (Fig. 1.3). The very small erectile body in the center expands into the large bulb (Fig. 1.3).

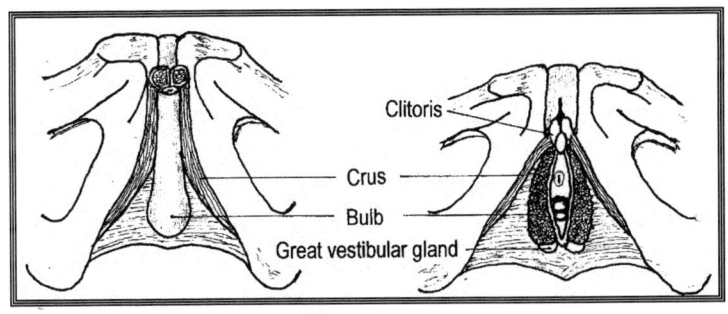

Figure 1.3

Although the body of Jasmine's clitoris is very tiny, it also contains three erectile bodies. Each erectile body (corpus cavernosum, clitoris) also tapers into a leg (crus, clitoris, Fig. 1.3) that is attached to the pubis bone. The thin central body divides into two long bulbs that flank the vestibule. The two small Bartholin's glands (great vestibular glands) are located under the bulbs.

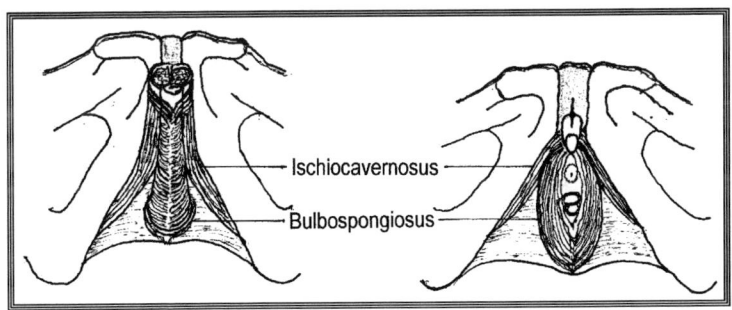

Figure 1.4

The muscles of the tapered legs of the erectile bodies of Kevin's penis and Jasmine's clitoris bear the same name (ischiocavernosus, Fig. 1.4). The name of the muscles of his penile bulb and her two clitoral bulbs are also the same (bulbospongiosus, Fig. 1.4).

3

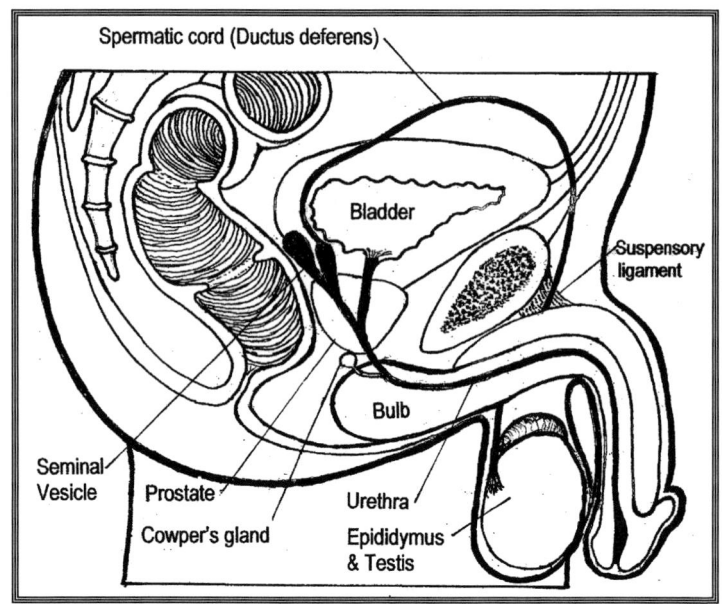

Figure 1.5

The diameter of an adult penis measures one to two inches (2.5-5 cm) or more (Fig. 1.5). Kevin owns an "average" organ of orgasm.

Jasmine appears to be very interested in the four outstanding secrets about the penis. But first, Kevin might not realize that his "average" organ is roughly ten inches long (25 cm). (Whoa, what a secret!)

Naturally, only five or six inches (13-15 cm) are visible, and the large bulb is hidden inside of his body (about 40 percent).

The second secret is that penis size is not related to Kevin's height, weight, or build, nor is it influenced by his nose, hands, or feet. It is also not based on his race, virility, or ability to give or receive sexual satisfaction – it is mainly determined by genetics.

4

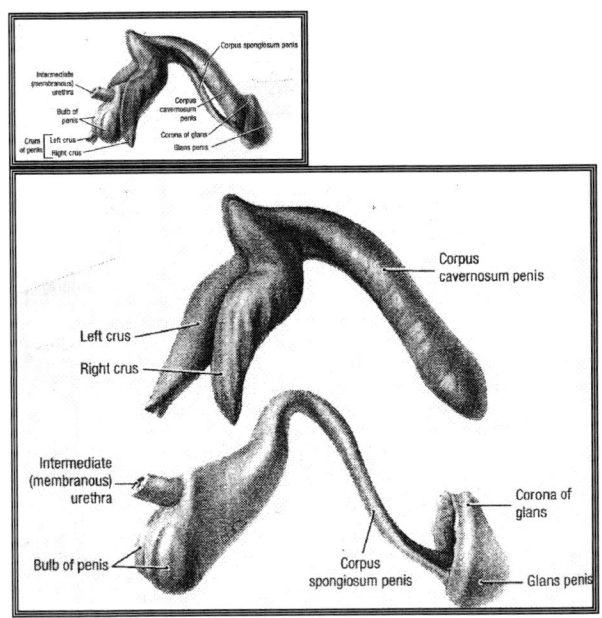

Figure1.6

The two erectile bodies (corpora cavernosum, penis) and legs (crura) are illustrated above the head (glans, penis), the tubelike body (corpus spongiosum), the bulb, and the enclosed urethra (Fig. 1.6).

The urethra is highly innervated and contains many smooth muscles. *The third secret is that during a penile erection, the "inverted pyramid" shape of Kevin's penis exposes his sensitive urethra to sexual stimulation.*

The head or glans, Latin for "acorn," and the rounded margin named the corona are packed with thousands of sensory receptors. The numerous nerves are enclosed under a thin layer of skin.

The fourth secret is that the most erogenous part of Kevin's erect penis is the thin-skinned glans, especially its highly sensitive corona.

The penile glans is covered by a soft, highly flexible fold of skin named the foreskin (prepuce). The foreskin may be removed shortly after birth in an operation called circumcision. Some people have it done for religious or cultural reasons and others for aesthetic preference or hygiene convenience.

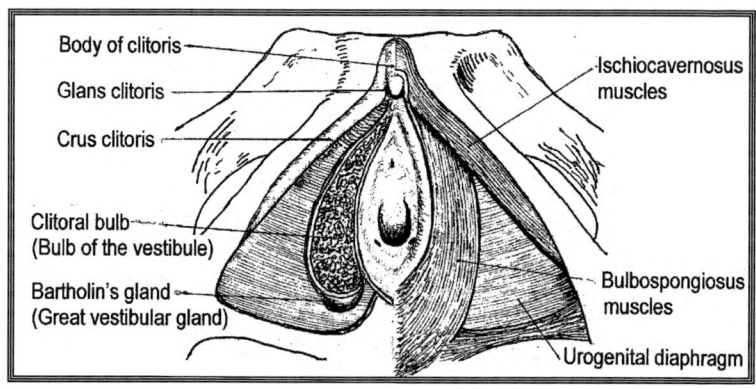

Figure 1.7

Kevin appears to be keenly interested in the four astonishing secrets about Jasmine's clitoris. The first secret is that the clitoris, Greek for "key," is called the female penis (coles femininus, Fig. 1.7).

The clitoris consists of the two bulbs (bulbs of the vestibule), the body and legs (crus, clitoris), and the head (glans, clitoris).

The glans and body of the clitoris are about an inch long (2.5 cm) and one-fourth of an inch (6 mm) in diameter, but these measurements may vary among individuals. The tiny glans contains thousands of

6

pressure receptors and nerve endings that are packed under a very fine layer of skin making it hypersensitive to touch, temperature, and pressure.

The second secret is that the most erogenous part of Jasmine's erect clitoris is the fine-skinned glans, especially the hypersensitive rounded margin called the corona.

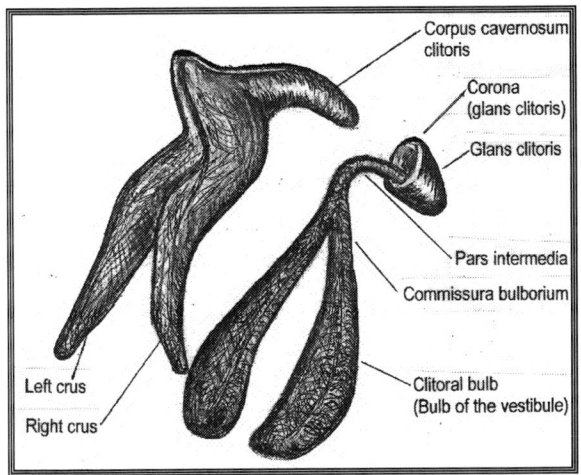

Figure 1.8

The two erectile bodies (corpora cavernosum, clitoris) and legs (crura, clitoris) are pictured above the head (glans, clitoris), the thin body (pars intermedia), the Y-shaped junction (commissura bulborium), and the bulbs of the clitoris (Fig. 1.8).

The clitoral bulbs are about three inches (7.6 cm) long and named the bulbs of the vestibule because of their location (Fig. 1.9).

The third secret is that the bulbs of the vestibule are, of course, parts of Jasmine's clitoris.

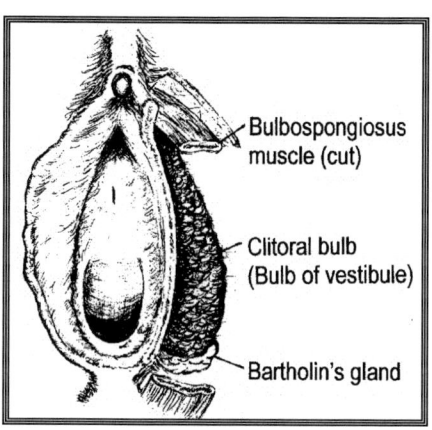

Bulbospongiosus muscle (cut)

Clitoral bulb (Bulb of vestibule)

Bartholin's gland

Figure 1.9

The fourth secret is that during a clitoral erection, the bulbs expand considerably, narrowing the entrance of the vagina to varying degrees. Jasmine's clitoral bulbs also become highly responsive to sexual stimulation (touch and pressure).

After learning these secrets, Jasmine says, "You know, Kev, I didn't realize that my clitoris went way down there! What secrets did you learn?"

"Secrets?" he replies. "I knew most of them, except for those two long things that are supposed to, ah, grip my organ. And it's nice to know, Jazzy, that my penis is at least – average."

"Let's go, Kevie," she says. "I can't wait for you to find out about the secrets of my three V's in the next chapter."

"Okay, Honey," Kevin replies. "I really need to learn the secrets of the vulva, vestibule, and especially, your vagina!"

2 Secrets of the Three V's

Jasmine's Vagina, Vestibule, and Vulva

Since his teens, Kevin has been intrigued but unfamiliar with the three V's. On this wedding night, however, it's imperative that Kevin learns the secrets of Jasmine's vagina, vestibule, and vulva.

The vulva, Latin for "covering," is the inverted triangular area that protects the urethra and vagina (Fig. 2.1). After puberty, the vulva is covered by spongy pubic hair.

The mysterious secret about the vulva is that the curly pubic hair harbors faint odorants (pheromones), a unique natural essence. Jasmine's pheromones may act as a powerful attractant that arouses Kevin's sexual desire.

At the apex of the vulva is the mons pubis, or "mountain" in Latin. When Jasmine is sexually aroused, the increased blood flow causes the mons to swell and become highly responsive to touch and pressure. The plump mons extends downward forming the outer or large lips (labia majora).

Like the mons, the outer lips also swell and become sensitive during sexual arousal. The large lips enclose the folds of delicate skin, the inner or little lips (labia minora).

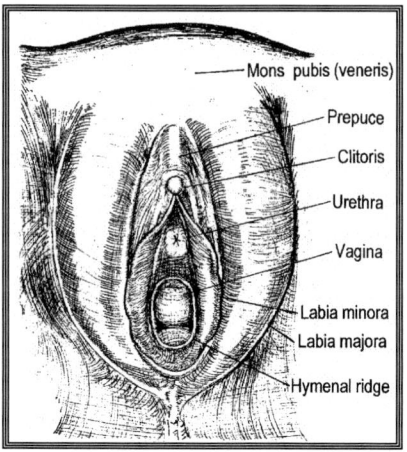

Figure 2.1

The thin inner lips fold above the body of the clitoris forming the hood or prepuce (the inside fold is attached at the glans). The inner lips also join below the clitoral body at the junction called the frenulum.

When Jasmine is sexually aroused, the rising inflow of blood causes the inner lips to enlarge slightly in diameter and could expand to more than twice their thickness. The blood flow also causes her pink inner lips to turn bright red, while others that are purplish red may become dark purple. The inner lips extend downward to enclose the vagina and the vestibule.

The vestibule is kept moist by its many mucous glands. This cavity is very delicate and sensitive (touch, pressure, and temperature). Below the clitoris is the slitlike orifice of the urethra (Fig. 2.2).

10

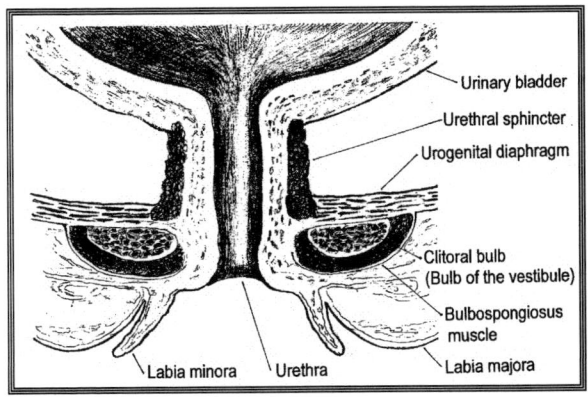

Figure 2.2

Jasmine appears to be the only one interested in the four unusual secrets about the urethra. First, the urethra is short – very short – only about one-and-a-half inches long (4 cm).

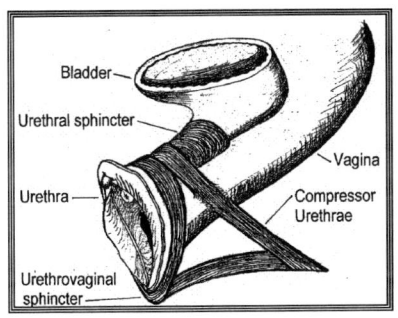

Figure 2.3

Second, the very short urethra is controlled and supported by at least five or six muscles.

The internal and external urethral sphincter muscles control the urethra only (Fig. 2.2). Two other muscles (compressor urethrae and urethrovaginalis sphincter, Fig. 2.3) compress both the urethra and the vagina. The strong pelvic floor muscles (levator ani) also control the urethra and the bladder.

Third, the urethra is partially fused to the upper front wall of the vagina. Sharing a joint common wall, Jasmine's urethra is very intimate with her vagina.

The urethra contains numerous smooth muscles and is highly innervated. *Fourth, when sexually aroused, Jasmine's urethra becomes erect and highly sensitive to sexual stimulation (touch and pressure).*

Emptying protective secretions into the urethra through ducts are the Skene's glands (para-urethral glands).

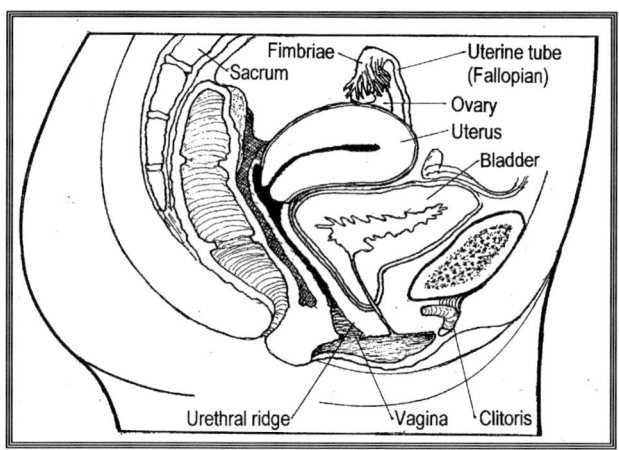

Figure 2.4

Below the urethra is the introitus (entrance) of the vagina (Fig. 2.4). The vagina, Latin meaning "sheath," is the strong, thin-walled muscular tube that connects the neck of the uterus (cervix) to the vestibule. The vagina empties various internal fluids, receives the penis during insemination, and delivers the newborn baby.

Apparently, Kevin is eager to uncover the five amazing secrets about the vagina. First, the introitus of Jasmine's vagina is located almost exactly where Kevin's penis exits his body.

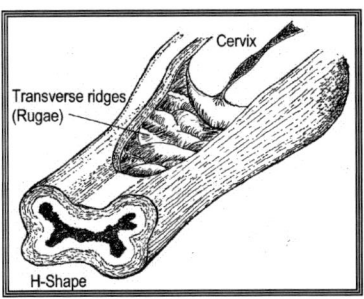

Figure 2.5

The upper wall of the vagina is about three to four inches long (8-10 cm), and the lower one is an inch longer. The walls usually lie close together like a flattened H-shaped tube (Fig. 2.5).

The interior is lined with rows of transverse ridges or rugae – soft folds of mucous membrane covered with scaly skin. Although the lining is mucous membrane, there are no mucous glands in the vagina.

Second, during sexual arousal, the massive inflow of blood alters the structure of the walls of the vagina by a unique process called transudation. The slick liquid (transudate) oozes through the semipermeable membrane of the vagina appearing on the walls like beads of sweat. Soon, the walls are flooded. The thin fluid acts as much as a cleaning solution and moisturizer as it does a lubricant.

A fold of mucous membrane called the hymen encloses the vagina. Typically, the small openings in the center of the hymen enlarge and become more irregular by sports activity, strenuous exercise, tampon usage, or pelvic exams. The hymen is worn away leaving the hymenal ring. *(Third, because Jasmine was an avid gymnast, she does not have an intact hymen.)*

Bulging out from the upper front wall is the wrinkled skin of the convex-shaped urethral ridge, which extends about two to three inches (5-8 cm) into the vagina. Since the vagina and the urethra share a joint common wall, the firm urethral ridge acts as a shield that protects the urethra.

When Jasmine is sexually aroused, her erect urethra may be accessed along the urethral ridge. *Fourth, while manipulating the wrinkled urethral ridge, Kevin might think that he is stimulating Jasmine's vagina, but the secret is that Jasmine's highly sensitive urethra is also being excited.*

Fifth, Jasmine's vagina is surrounded and strengthened by at least seven muscles (or groups of muscles). The two muscles that compress the vagina and urethra (compressor urethrae and urethrovaginalis sphincter) are shown in Figure 2.3 (page 11).

Figure 2.6 illustrates the other five muscles. The uppermost group stretches from the rectum to the bladder (rectovesicalis). Next are the front parts of the PC muscles that pull the middle of the vagina towards the pubis bone (pubovaginalis).

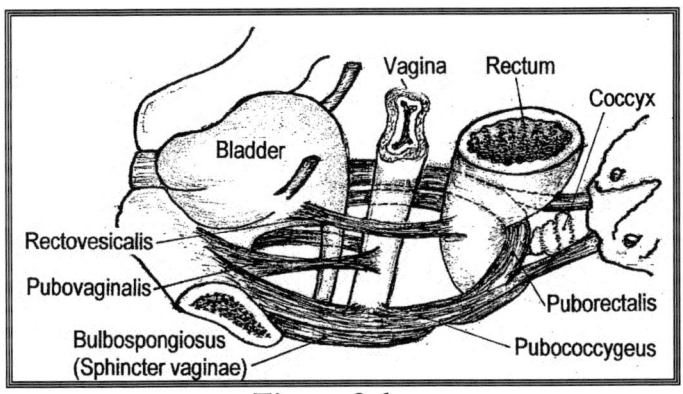

Figure 2.6

Below them are the potent pubococcygeus (PC) muscles (of the levator ani) that tighten all the way from the pubis bone to the spinal column. The puborectalis (of the PC) forms a sling around the vagina and rectum. And in the lower vagina are the strong muscles (bulbospongiosus) of the two clitoral bulbs.

The muscles help to hold a developing baby during pregnancy and to powerfully push it out at childbirth. They are instantly activated during a hard cough, a healthy sneeze, or a convulsive orgasm.

Because harmful microbes can enter Jasmine's body through her vagina, there are three defenses to combat them. The first defense is acidity (pH 3.8-5.2). The scaly lining of the vagina contains large amounts of glycogen. The vagina's normal resident Doderlein's bacilli or lactobacillus can breakdown the glycogen forming lactic acid.

To protect the vaginal lining from acidity, the second defense is provided by various substances (some alkaline) that are constantly flowing in and out of the vagina. Mucus and fluids flow from the ovaries, oviducts, uterus, and from the vagina itself. The sticky mucus traps the entering microbes for removal. The endometrium or unused uterus lining also takes days to flow out during menstruation.

Jasmine's third defense is her potent immune system. Millions of white blood cells (leukocytes and macrophages) diligently patrol the vagina and gobble up harmful microbes as well as many unsuspecting sperm cells.

The lower ends of the vagina and urethra are held in place by ligaments and two strong diaphragms. The lower vagina also contains numerous nerve endings making it highly sensitive to touch, pressure, and temperature. The upper vagina contains very few nerves but may respond to pressure.

First to react to this new information is Jasmine. "I'll bet, Kev, that you didn't know how muscle-bound my vagina was, right?" she asks.

"Yes, Jazzy, I didn't know," he answers.

Hugging him, Jasmine says, "Now, Kevie, remember where everything is and don't rush in – always wait for lots of lubrication!"

"All right, Honey, but I want to learn how to get it up and keep it up," Kevin replies. "I'm going to look for the secrets of erection, emission, and ejaculation."

chapter

3 Secrets of the Three E's

Erection, Emission, and Ejaculation

Jasmine and Kevin might not know that the secrets of the three E's are hidden in the most potent sex organ in the body – the human brain.

At the "heart" of the complex nervous system is the brain. Not only does it control Kevin's and Jasmine's vital, everyday functions and physical actions, the brain enables them to read books, build computers, and to be human. The brain is also the home of the mind and, of course, where sex really happens.

The brain looks large and rather heavy, but it only weighs about three pounds (1.5 kg). Although the brain is merely two percent of the body mass, it receives twenty percent of the body's blood, oxygen, and energy output. This means that the brain demands sixteen times more blood, oxygen, and energy than any other body part or its tissues will rapidly begin to die.

The brain performs its job with highly specialized nerve cells or neurons. Neurobiologists estimate that there are more than 100 billion neurons in the brain.

And deep within the center of gray and white matter is the most significant part of the brain, the hypothalamus, called the hypo-T for short.

The hypo-T (a region of the diencephalon) is part of the brain stem and located at the lower limits of the brain, way back of the sinuses, and just above the roof of the mouth (Fig. 3.1).

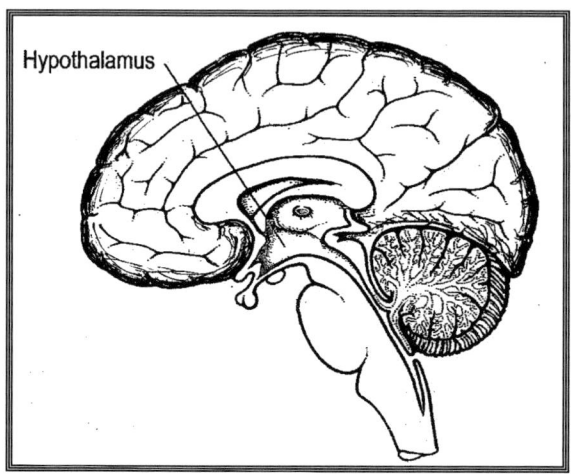

Figure 3.1

Although this vital part of the brain weighs almost nothing at four grams and is less than one percent of the brain mass, the unfamiliar secret is that anatomy books refer to the hypothalamus as the "brain in the brain" and even the "head honcho" of the brain.

To understand its importance, the "brain in the brain" is the major link between the nervous system and the endocrine glands (hormones). The hypo-T consists of more than a dozen nuclei (specialized glands).

Each nucleus produces unique regulating hormones and chemical messengers (neurotransmitters). The nuclei activate and control the adrenal glands, ovaries, testes, thymus gland, thyroid glands, and others in the body. Some nuclei regulate the body's biological clock, while others manage the body's hunger center, thirst center, sleep center, and, of course, the sex center.

The "head honcho" of the brain also functions as the body's main regulatory center. The hypo-T activates and controls Jasmine's and Kevin's autonomic or automatic nervous system (ANS) and its main divisions, the sympathetic nervous system (SNS) and parasympathetic nervous system (PNS). Utilizing the ANS, the hypo-T is in charge of the body's temperature, heart and breathing rates, blood pressure, digestion, metabolic rate, and homeostasis (internal environment).

In concert with the other higher cerebral centers, the hypo-T makes it possible for Jasmine and Kevin to participate in expressions of aggression, pain, pleasure, rage, and behaviors related to sexual arousal, including the three E's: erection, emission, and ejaculation.

Kevin is eager to learn the three notable secrets about erections. The first secret is that Kevin's organ of orgasm can experience not one, not two, but three types of erections, and so can Jasmine's clitoris.

The first type is the reflex or reflexogenic erection that is activated by the reflex capability of the spinal cord; it is similar to a knee jerk. A sharp tap to the

19

ligament under the kneecap speeds sensory impulses to the spinal cord that flashes reflex signals to the thigh muscle, pulling the lower leg forward in a knee jerk.

Similarly, sexual stimulation of the organ of orgasm speeds sensory signals to the erection center (located in the lower spinal cord). The erection center flashes reflex impulses through the parasympathetic nerves (PNS) to the organ, initiating a reflex erection that could be called a "clitoris jerk" for Jasmine or a "penis jerk" for Kevin.

The second type is the mental or psychogenic erection that is initiated by what Kevin or Jasmine sees, imagines, smells, hears, or touches (other than genitals). Kevin responds well to what he sees and touches, whereas Jasmine is mainly influenced by what she imagines, smells, and touches. The higher cerebral centers and hypo-T flash signals to the erection center via the PNS nerves to the clitoris or penis initiating a psychogenic erection.

And the third type is Jasmine's NCT or nocturnal clitoral tumescence (swelling) and Kevin's nocturnal penile tumescence (NPT). Jasmine and Kevin may experience four to six rapid eye movement (REM) sleep phases in a typical night's rest of seven to nine hours. Kevin's hypo-T initiates an NPT event during each REM sleep phase, while Jasmine's hypo-T causes an NCT episode.

The second secret about erections is that during a typical night, Jasmine's clitoris or Kevin's penis can be erect for a total time of one to three-and-a-half hours. (Wow, what a secret!) At times, Jasmine and Kevin may awaken with an erection. This occurs because they were in a REM sleep phase when awakened.

Research urologists have determined that the increased oxygen and blood flow during NPT and NCT episodes may prevent too much collagen from forming in the erectile tissues of the clitoris and penis. They know that excessive collagen could cause increased fiber formation in the erectile tissues that may lead to tissue-cell death and loss of erectile function.

And the third secret about erections is that Jasmine's clitoral and Kevin's penile erections are similar.

When the organ of orgasm is lax and soft, or flaccid, the hypo-T maintains the sympathetic nerve signals (SNS) keeping the organ's supply arteries narrow. With low blood inflow, the organ remains flaccid (Fig. 3.2).

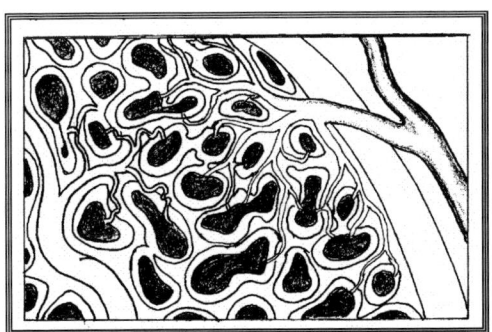

Figure 3.2

In the latent or filling phase, the hypo-T activates the PNS nerve signals enlarging the organ's arteries. Blood gushes into the spongy cavities of the erectile bodies, but the organ of orgasm is only slightly swollen and the erection is still hidden.

During the short swelling phase, the blood inflow rapidly increases to four to ten times the flaccid rate, causing the spongy cavities to expand. The draining veins are compressed between the surrounding sheaths and the rapidly expanding erectile bodies. This effectively traps the blood in the organ of orgasm (Fig. 3.3).

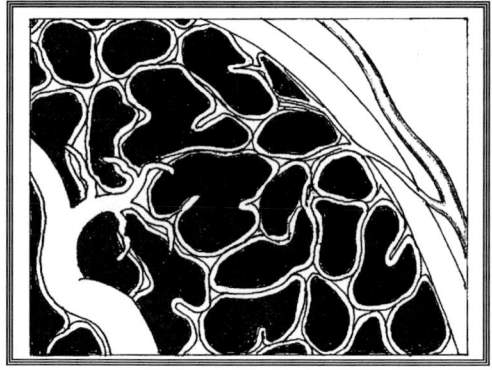

Figure 3.3

As the blood inflow diminishes, the organ of orgasm is completely engorged with blood during the full erection phase. The organ's volume of blood could be up to eight times greater than when it is lax and soft.

The organ (clitoris or penis) becomes hard and stiff during the rigid erection phase because of the tightening of the muscles enclosing the erectile bodies and their strong legs. The inflow of blood is very low and blood outflow is almost zero.

In the deflating phase, the hypo-T activates the SNS nerve signals narrowing the organ's arteries. With restricted blood inflow and increasing blood outflow, the organ of orgasm loses its stiffness and becomes flaccid.

Emission and ejaculation are actions that occur during Kevin's orgasm. After receiving maximum sexual stimulation, Kevin's hypo-T speeds SNS nerve signals to various organs for the production of semen (milky fluid containing sperm cells).

The complex process of emission begins with the two pea-shaped Cowper's glands, as their thick fluid cleanses and lubricates the urethra. The prostate gland contributes a slightly acidic liquid. From the testicles, the spermatic cords supply a grayish fluid containing between 200 million and 600 million sperm! The two nutrition pouches (seminal vesicles) supply a volume of nutrient-rich (fructose) fluid that is needed for sperm survival.

Ejaculation is a reflex that transports the semen out of Kevin's body. Although the reaction is quite complex, Kevin finds it rather easy to produce.

He could experience a spontaneous ejaculation, even in the absence of an erection. Rapid or premature ejaculations just happen. Kevin may even have a "wet dream" while asleep. There are times, however, when Kevin wants to ejaculate, but it does not matter what he does, how hard or long he tries – an ejaculation simply does not occur.

Kevin's personal secret is that an ejaculation could be triggered by stimulating – individually or collectively – the numerous nerves of the urethra and penis, especially the sensitive glans and its highly sensitive corona. There may be other ways of inducing Kevin's ejaculation.

When Kevin attains the peak of psychic and physical sexual stimulation, the hypo-T sends signals to the various organs of emission. Immediately after sensing the fullness of emission, Kevin experiences an ejaculation – the sudden release of built-up sexual tension.

Kevin's lower body could shudder from the involuntary, pulsating compressions (about one to two per second) of the muscles of the urethra, the two erectile body legs, the anal sphincter, and the large bulb. The semen could shoot out a great distance in wavelike spurts or might only ooze out over the glans. The ejaculation completes his orgasm.

Kevin might not be familiar with the two awesome secrets about Jasmine's orgasm. First, Jasmine's climax could be initiated by stimulating – individually or collectively – the sensitive urethra (along the wrinkled urethral ridge in the vagina) and the clitoris, especially its hypersensitive glans and excitable bulbs. There may be other ways of bringing about Jasmine's orgasm.

The other awesome secret is that during her orgasm, the contractions of the muscles of Jasmine's elongated clitoral bulbs are similar to the compressions of the muscles of Kevin's penile bulb,

24

during his ejaculation. In this book, the climactic reaction of the muscles of Jasmine's elongated clitoral bulbs is called the "orgasmic reflex."

As soon as Jasmine attains the maximum of psychic and physical sexual sensations, she feels the sudden discharge of built-up sexual tension.

Jasmine's whole lower body may quiver from the involuntary, pulsating contractions (about one to three per second) of the anal sphincter muscles, the pelvic floor and PC muscles, the four other vaginal muscles, the ringed muscles encircling the urethra and vagina, and then the orgasmic reflex – the sharp, equally rapid spasms of the strong muscles of the elongated clitoral bulbs. The orgasmic reflex completes Jasmine's orgasm.

At this point, Jasmine exclaims, "You know, Kev, I've often wondered how my clitoris gets an erection, but I didn't know that it was so complicated!"

"Of course, Jazzy, an erection is simply the genital psychovasoneuromuscular event that is synchronized by the hypothalamus, neurotransmitters, and regulating hormones," Kevin replies.

"All right, Kevin, please don't get technical with me," says Jasmine. "Besides, I found out what's happening to me during my orgasmic reflex!"

Then Kevin says, "Don't worry, Honey, because I think I know how to get it up and keep it up, guaranteed!"

"Okay, Kev," says Jasmine. "But before we get started, let's take a look at the secrets of our libidos."

4

Secrets of Sex Drive

Kevin's and Jasmine's Sex Drives

The fascinating secrets about sex drive are hidden in the hypothalamus, the "head honcho" of the brain that is in charge of the hunger, thirst, sleep, and sex centers. The secrets of Jasmine's and Kevin's sex centers began at conception.

When Kevin was conceived, the nucleus of his father's *male* sperm cell contained the smaller Y-sex chromosome and its SRY gene's blueprint to form testicles instead of ovaries. But he still needed some special hormones to become a regular guy.

Ten weeks after Kevin's conception, the hypo-T sent regulating hormones and chemical messengers to his testes to begin producing androgens (any substance that promotes masculinization). The principal androgen is testosterone. Eight weeks later, his testosterone level was proportionately equal to that of an adult male, causing the primitive sex organ to develop into his penis.

The testes were directed to make a steady supply of androgens, at least until Kevin was born. Strangely, after the great escape from his mother's womb, his testosterone output was drastically reduced to very low levels during boyhood. At puberty, the hypo-T reawakened his testes, and his androgen secretion increased to eight times the levels Kevin made as a boy.

During adolescence, the masculinizing hormones advanced tissue development in all areas of Kevin's body. Androgens were responsible for his broad shoulders, narrow waist and hips, and deep voice. Testosterone also caused the growth of his Adam's apple, prostate gland, and potent reproductive system.

Kevin grew for a longer period of time than Jasmine, which resulted in his longer bones, greater height, and bigger brain. Androgens amplified his bone and muscle volume, but cut body fat to only 13 to 15 percent. From puberty, the hypo-T directs a steady stream of these vital steroid hormones that continues for the rest of Kevin's life.

As a young man, Kevin's hypo-T also causes the adrenal glands (located in the fat pads above the kidneys) to secrete scant amounts of androgens. These hormones provide an extra boost to Kevin's libido and are responsible for secondary sexual characteristics, such as facial, armpit, and pubic hair growth.

The combination of a larger brain and testosterone makes Kevin aggressive, assertive, and a risk taker. He could always be wondering about how things like watches, guns, or cars work, but might not have a clue about how people work. He can excel in math, science, or medicine, but could have difficulty trying to communicate.

Kevin could display a lot of talent in music or creativity in art, but may not have the social skills to understand Jasmine's mind and emotions. He has very good visual-spatial skills and finds it easy to park cars, dive nuclear submarines, or pilot jumbo jets. Testosterone drives Kevin to be highly attracted to Jasmine, although he might have difficulty trying to be intimate with her.

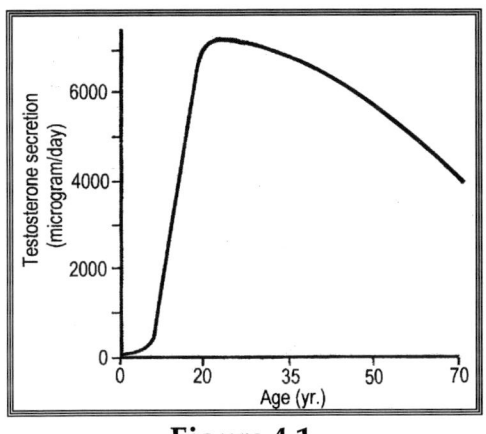

Figure 4.1

Since testosterone appears to influence Kevin's sex drive, the hormone's secretion curve could be a perfect picture of his lifetime libido (Fig. 4.1). Now in his twenties, the highest lifetime levels must have had something to do with his meeting and marrying Jasmine. When Kevin gets to middle age, he might sense a gradual, hard-to-detect decrease in his sex drive.

Unfortunately, Kevin's libido could take a steep slide during his forties and fifties – the dreaded midlife crisis. Not to worry, because he will still have enough of his sex hormones to "get the job done." When finally eligible for Medicare in his sixties, Kevin's testosterone tank may be half full or half empty, either scenario won't be good. But Kevin will still have enough of his manly hormones, although, from then on, the frequency of his sexual episodes might be affected.

Kevin's daily production of androgens is complex. Simply stated, however, the hypo-T causes the release of testosterone to rise and fall with his unique biological clock.

Kevin might not realize that his testosterone secretion level secretly swings to a peak in the morning, drops off in the afternoon, and may rise again at night. (Hmmm, is this the key to his daily sex drive?)

Androgens are also needed for the production of sperm cells. Daily, the hypo-T also sends regulating hormones and chemical messengers to his testes to form sperm germ cells (spermatogonia), rough count: 120 million! Each sperm germ cell's job is to divide twice, producing four new half-cells, two of each sex, and each with its own unique genetic makeup.

Each newly formed sperm cell, with the aid of testosterone, takes almost three months to develop (spermiogenesis) into a fully mature, motile sperm cell (spermatozoon).

Also, Kevin might not know that every day, on average, about 300 million sperm secretly reach maturity in his two testicles! (Incredible and some guys may mature even more!)

But aside from his androgens, astronomical sperm bank, and hypo-T, Kevin's sex drive is also influenced by the state of his body, mind, and spirit.

It's no secret that the greatest enemy of Kevin's libido is fatigue, brought on by the lack of sleep, overwork, stress, or poor nutrition. He might not be interested in sex because of substance abuse, cardio or vascular diseases, or even some essential medication. Other culprits could include aging, obesity, or even the lack of nighttime erections.

Psychological factors such as poor self-image, sexual inhibition, or performance anxiety could affect Kevin's desire for sex. Other factors may include the lack of sexual information, unsatisfactory sexual communication issues, disappointing sexual experiences, or the failure to seek help for sexual or erectile dysfunction.

Spiritual bliss could rely on contentment in his marriage. Kevin's marital happiness may depend upon a healthy sex drive and great sexual satisfaction with Jasmine. While acknowledging God as the head of his marriage *(others may look to some other power)*, Kevin makes a lifetime commitment to care for, trust, respect, have faith in, and love his wife Jasmine.

Now married, the macho man Kevin is supposed to have a great and inexhaustible sex drive. Isn't this why he will be expected to be the leader in sexual affairs? But are the secrets of Jasmine's sex drive quite different or more similar?

Upon Jasmine's conception, the nucleus of her father's *female* sperm was structured with the X-sex chromosome and its genetic blueprint to form ovaries. After only five weeks of life, Jasmine's newly forming ovaries may have already contained some 200 primordial germ egg cells (oogonia) that began proliferating by a super-rapid multiplication process called mitosis.

Jasmine is shocked when she discovers the incredible secrets about her ovaries. Only three weeks later, Jasmine's embryonic ovaries were teeming with 600,000 primary oocytes as the hyper-activity continued! At six months after conception, her fetal ovaries were bursting with 6 million to 7 million primary oocytes!

(From this peak, the number of oocytes reduced rapidly by a process called atresia. When Jasmine was born, her ovaries may have contained up to 2 million oocytes, more than enough for a lifetime. The steady reduction continued. By puberty, her ovaries contained some 30,000 to 40,000 now called primary follicles. Of these, only 400 to 500 may reach maturity.)

Ten weeks after conception, the hypo-T sent chemical messengers and regulating hormones to her embryonic ovaries to also begin producing estrogen and progesterone. The X-sex chromosome's genetic blueprint and Jasmine's hormones caused the genital tubercle to transform into her tiny clitoris.

It also appears that Jasmine is very interested in the three extraordinary secrets about estrogen. Firstly, as Jasmine developed in the womb, the hormones made her brain cells dense.

Unlike Kevin's testes, which provided a steady stream of androgens, Jasmine's ovaries furnished a variable amount of hormones. After birth, the hormone secretion was drastically reduced to very low levels during her childhood – until puberty.

During adolescence, the hypo-T prompted her teenage ovaries to secrete high levels of estrogen and progesterone, about twenty times more than when she was a child. Between the ages of eleven and thirteen years, the hormones assisted in Jasmine's rapid body growth. But early sealing of the long bones stopped her growth at about fourteen to sixteen years of age.

Secondly, estrogen secretly enables Jasmine to easily store fat. On average, her body fat may be 25 to 27 percent, almost twice as much as Kevin.

Jasmine's increased secretion of hormones also helped to form a larger and wider pelvis, as her external genitals enlarged. The ovaries, oviducts, uterus, and vagina doubled in size as her reproductive system developed.

Estrogen and progesterone make a woman a woman. Estrogen softens the skin and progesterone makes it warm. The increased level of estrogen and progesterone also began to develop the tissues of the breasts and the growth of the extensive ductile system (mammary glands) as Jasmine transformed into a young woman. Collectively, the development was ultimately responsible for the characteristic appearance of her mature female breasts.

Thirdly, estrogen secretly developed a thicker bundle of transverse fibers (corpus callosum). The larger connection enables Jasmine to use both sides of her brain at the same time and, therefore, to multitask.

The dense, well-connected brain cells sharpen the social and relationship skills that enable Jasmine to understand and recognize her emotions as well as those of others. Although the hormone secretion fluctuates throughout her reproductive life, the average level remains high.

During each ovarian cycle, Jasmine's hypo-T regulates the level of estrogen and progesterone to rise and fall in a coordinated effort to develop and nurture a single mature egg (ovum). And Jasmine's peak libido usually appears just before ovulation.

Then, Jasmine uncovers the startling secret that her sex drive may be just as high at other times, because like Kevin's libido, her desire is also fueled by androgens.

The hypo-T directs her adrenal glands to secrete a scant but potent androgen supply that plays a vital role in Jasmine's lifetime sex drive and other sexual behaviors. The adrenal androgens also promote secondary sexual characteristics, such as hair growth on her face, armpits, pubic region, and lower arms and legs.

The adrenals also secrete small amounts of estrogen and progesterone. Her adrenal glands are an important source of these hormones after menopause.

At menopause, Jasmine's once rich supply of estrogen, progesterone, and ovum from her ovaries will finally be too low for reproduction.

But aside from her hormones and hypo-T, Jasmine needs to feel good about her appearance, for herself and for Kevin. She needs to maintain a high energy level by keeping active.

Jasmine's health and other factors could be exactly the same as those experienced by Kevin and may significantly affect her sex drive. Spiritual bliss can also depend upon contentment in her marriage. Jasmine's marital happiness could depend upon a healthy sex drive and great sexual satisfaction with Kevin. While also acknowledging God as the head of her marriage, Jasmine makes a lifetime commitment to care for, trust, respect, have faith in, and love her husband Kevin.

After a long sigh, Jasmine says, "Oh, Kevin, are you serious? I can't imagine that your body matures 300 million sperm everyday! Now I know why you've always been after me for – you know what."

"I always thought, Jazzy, that you only made one egg a month," Kevin replies. "And I finally found out why you can do so many things at the same time, and I can't."

"Well, I'm glad that you're paying attention," Jasmine says, rubbing him. "Now hurry up, Kevie, so that you can learn the secrets of arousal, you know, how to turn me on!"

"Okay, Honey," Kevin replies. "Let's find out the secrets of prolonged petting."

5

Secrets of the First Phase

Foreplay or Prolonged Petting

It's no secret that foreplay is the universal prelude to sex. And Jasmine and Kevin begin their passionate lovemaking by employing the largest and heaviest sex organ in the human body – the skin. Jasmine can't imagine that Kevin's thin skin weighs as much as 11 pounds (5 kg) and can be rolled out to cover the front door of their new house!

Essentially, Kevin and Jasmine are "naked apes" covered by fine body hair. The covering of skin, hair, nails, various glands, muscles, and nerves (integumentary system) is monitored by the somatic nervous system containing more than five million receptors.

A sensory receptor is simply a nerve ending that detects a certain sensation. The five senses are touch, pain, pressure, warmth, and cold, and each has its own sensory receptor.

When it comes to Kevin's highly sensitive body parts, many types of nerve endings are found on his tender tongue, lips, and feet. The numerous receptors are also found on his fingers and penis (Fig. 5.1). Jasmine's supersensory receptors are found on her luscious lips and tongue, dainty fingers and feet, and her exquisite breasts and clitoris.

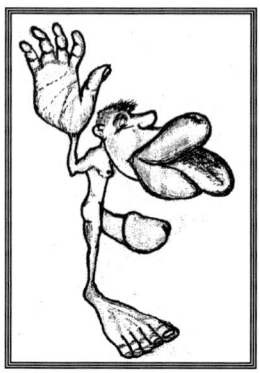

Figure 5.1

Skillful skin-to-skin contact naturally adds to feelings of pleasure and sexual arousal. When Kevin uses a finger to stimulate an exposed area on her body, the feathery touch prompts a ticklish sensation. Jasmine giggles and squirms, while at the same time, becoming sexually aroused.

Now that they're married, foreplay is effortless because it is anticipated and expected. Jasmine knows that Kevin is always "in the mood" for love and doesn't need any of the preliminaries. But Jasmine might not be as ready because of her hypo-T and higher cerebral centers.

To get ready for this wedding night, Jasmine needs to be settled and content. Her "emotional brain" might still be thinking about the wedding arrangements that failed to follow her plans or how she really meant to decorate their new house.

Foreplay can't proceed until Jasmine is able to set her unresolved items aside (at least in her mind's eye), and she is calm and relaxed.

Has Kevin been doing a good job by keeping Jasmine happy? Is he continuing to talk to her about any unresolved issues? Is Kevin paying enough attention to meet her needs? Does Jasmine feel neglected, and if so, by how much?

Before anything can happen in the honeymoon suite, Jasmine has to feel safe and secure. Has the "Do Not Disturb" sign been posted and the door double-locked? Are the drapes drawn and the lights turned down or off? Where are the cell phones? When everything is secure, they can finally get started.

There could be an easy-to-find trail of clothing leading to the comfortable bed. Jasmine and Kevin are partially clothed or may already be comfortably naked. They embrace and express their feelings of intimacy, tenderness, and love, by using their soft, luscious lips. Their mouths are avenues of pleasure and are used for kissing, which is both an oral and erotic activity.

Their kisses reveal that Kevin and Jasmine have crossed over from puppy love to sexual affection. The short, tender kisses extend to the long, lingering ones that lead into the deep French kiss.

This passionate kiss involves tongue probing of the insides of the mouth or mutual tongue sucking, the universal inborn response. In the exchange of saliva, they could sense the presence of pheromones, which may be responsible for the erogenous sensations felt during deep kissing.

Kevin's kissing edges around to sucking, nibbling, and playful biting of Jasmine's ear lobes. Moving lower, he leaves a trail of hickie marks on her neck and shoulders. His hands gently caress Jasmine's super-soft breasts. Kevin's contact with her smooth breasts certainly creates a two-way charge of foreplay excitement.

Just the sight of her beautiful breasts is enough to cause his pupils to open wide. Obviously, Jasmine's exquisite breasts are the essence of her femininity, and there's nothing quite like them on her body. Kevin has to remind himself that the size of her perfectly shaped breasts has nothing to do with their sensitivity, especially the nipples, which he adores.

While kissing and fondling her swelling breasts, Kevin arrives at the tense nipples. Nipple kissing advances to sucking, then to suckling, the lifesaving behavior that Kevin instinctively learned while still in his mother's womb. To suckle, the sensory nerves at the base of the nipple are pinched or squeezed by the lips or tongue while sucking.

The unexpected secret is that Kevin's suckling is prompting Jasmine's higher cerebral centers and hypo-T to release oxytocin into her blood stream.

The stimulating hormone contracts the muscles surrounding Jasmine's mammary glands, contributing to their firmness. Oxytocin could also alter the contour of her breasts and may increase their size by as much as twenty to thirty percent.

Jasmine's arousal advances as the hypo-T raises her heart rate, blood pressure, and breathing rate. Her body temperature increases as the upper mons sweats, swells, and becomes highly sensitive to the touch. The surging inflow of blood causes the large outer lips to swell and flatten out toward the thighs, exposing the delicate inner lips that could double in thickness and change from pink to a bright or darker red.

The body of Jasmine's clitoris may double in thickness and lengthen slightly. The glans tries to rise as it tugs on the highly flexible hood. The very fine-skinned glans also becomes hypersensitive, making any direct contact there feel more like an irritation than an erotic touch.

The thin, muscular walls of Jasmine's vagina begin to thicken, as the inner walls swell around the neck of the uterus. The massive blood inflow induces transudation, as a copious volume of slick fluid appears like sweat that soon floods her vaginal walls. The expanding clitoral bulbs lengthen and press down against the two small Bartholin's glands that release slippery secretions at the introitus of her vagina.

The increasing body heat also manifests itself in the sex flush (maculopapular rash) appearing on Jasmine's neck and upper chest area. The gooseflesh could spread down to her back, upper buttocks, and around to the abdomen. It looks like Jasmine is responding well to Kevin's petting activities.

Since Kevin is ready but Jasmine may need more time, prolonged foreplay is usually recommended. While extending this phase may have its merits, there could be some potential problems.

For instance, Kevin's positive feedback system, monitored by the hypo-T and higher cerebral centers, automatically advances his penile erection and orgasmic potential.

There are two precautionary secrets about prolonged foreplay. First, during his efforts to arouse Jasmine, Kevin might not realize that he is also stimulating himself and could "lose it" by ejaculating rapidly or prematurely.

Meanwhile, extending foreplay advances Jasmine's clitoral erection and the enlargement of her two clitoral bulbs. *Second, the extended time could cause a much greater expansion of Jasmine's elongated clitoral bulbs, making Kevin's initial penetration difficult to varying degrees and, at times, almost impossible. And Kevin might not be aware of this secret, as well.*

With her head on a soft pillow, Jasmine looks up at Kevin, who is kneeling below her. After she brings her knees up, he slowly spreads her legs exposing the vestibule.

When her delicate inner lips separate, Kevin picks up the erotic scent that is Jasmine's unique feminine essence. The vaginal fluids may contain pheromones possessing aphrodisiac qualities, and Kevin finds it quite pleasant and sexually stimulating.

Using his longest finger, Kevin tests Jasmine's readiness. As it slides along the smooth surfaces of her delicate inner lips, he carefully searches for the shallow indentation of Jasmine's vagina and its abundant fluids. The slick vaginal liquids are necessary for pleasant massaging sensations.

Gently inserting his finger into the horizontal, slitlike introitus of Jasmine's vagina, the first thing that Kevin feels is the hymenal ring and then the beginning of the firm convex urethral ridge. Pinching in on the sides of his finger are Jasmine's vaginal walls, which are backed by her two swollen elongated clitoral bulbs (Fig. 5.2).

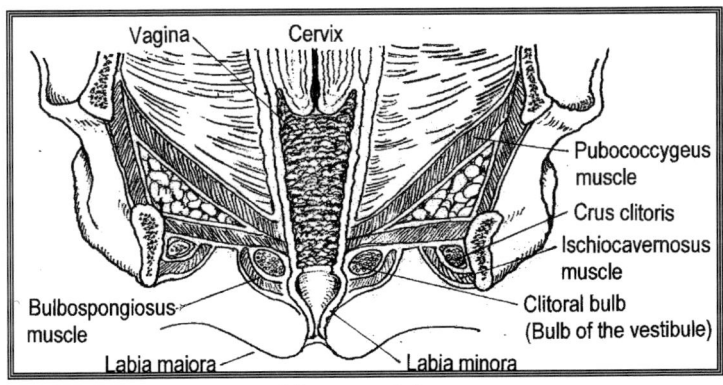

Figure 5.2

As Kevin slowly slides his finger in, it rides up and around the wrinkled urethral ridge. And if his finger is long enough, it touches the soft ball-like appendage of the cervix that acts like a bumper at the upper end of Jasmine's vagina.

Anxiously, Kevin is worrying about how his bulbous penis is going to penetrate into Jasmine's very narrow vagina. Perhaps he has just taken too much time. Jasmine's vagina, however, is extremely tight, well lubricated, and ready for sexplay.

First to speak is Jasmine, "Boy, Kev, am I glad that you finally found out about my clitoral bulbs and that they're the reason why it gets so tight down there."

"I know, Jazzy," Kevin replies. "Now I know why I'm going to have a hard time just trying to get it in."

"Well, Kevin, let's get it in and stop chatting," says Jasmine.

"Who, me?" Kevin answers. "Look who's talking. Let's find the secrets of sexplay — that's next. Ah, what did you just say, Honey?"

"Kevin, I said, let's get it in, already!"

chapter

6 Secrets of the Second Phase

Sensational Sexplay

During Kevin's passionate foreplay activities, the scrotum sack has pulled his testicles up close to his body. Even his nipples have become erect. Kevin's higher cerebral centers and hypo-T have steadily advanced his organ to the rigid erection phase. Kevin appears to be ready for sexplay.

While Kevin is positioned between Jasmine's outstretched legs, a clear drop of mucus appears out of the urethra and hangs on the end of his penis like a heavy raindrop. The mucoid liquid has just arrived from his two tiny Cowper's glands.

The slightly alkaline fluid neutralizes any acidic leftovers in the urethra. The slippery solution also forms a protective coating for the millions of sperm cells that are getting ready to make a small explosion out of the urethra, as little as 200 million, to perhaps as many as 600 million! Kevin is finally ready.

Kevin uses his penis to gently probe for Jasmine's upper vaginal introitus and is extra careful not to slip into the lower one. After locating the shallow indentation, Kevin gently nudges his penis in. As it enters the horizontal slit-like introitus, Kevin's penile glans is "crushed" when it meets Jasmine's convex urethral ridge bulging on top and her swollen clitoral bulbs on the sides. To Kevin, it feels like the glans of his penis is being choked down, literally, to the size of a No. 2 pencil!

Because Jasmine's vagina is so unyielding, only the front part of his penile glans can get in, and Kevin can only make very shallow thrusting motions. With each thrust, he takes a deep breath and presses forward a few millimeters at a time. While withdrawing, Kevin tries to gather momentum for another very short stroke forward. It is extremely slow going, and he is careful not to force anything that might be painful to Jasmine or to him.

Gradually, the taut ring of Jasmine's vagina stretches and allows more and more of his penile glans in. After what feels like a very long time for Kevin, the bulbous glans of his penis finally makes its way into her vagina.

Sighing in relief, Kevin has a marvelous, heart-warming feeling because Jasmine's vagina feels like such a wonderful place. He is overcome by the fantastic sensation of the smooth, wet, and warm sheath tightly holding on to his penis. Kevin thinks that he has finally found what it means to be intimate with Jasmine, to merge and to become one with her. He is soaring "high like an eagle" in a make-believe world of his own, when suddenly, he feels the familiar buildup of an oncoming orgasm!

Kevin is petrified and wants to escape, but Jasmine's wrapped legs have him trapped! Taking a deep breath, he holds it and squeezes, but it's too late! After only a brief period of sexplay, Kevin feels the sudden release of an explosive ejaculation. Because of the euphoria that Kevin felt after initially entering Jasmine's vagina, his lack of experience, or his normal reaction timing, Kevin climaxes rapidly and unexpectedly.

(The predictable secret is that a rapid ejaculation occurs easily. Perhaps, Kevin wasn't extra careful, especially after his initial penetration. But on this wedding night, Kevin holds off the premature ejaculation and gets a second chance.)

Kevin panics and stops all movement! He wants to pull out to escape, but Jasmine's legs have him trapped! Taking a deep breath, he holds it and squeezes, as the orgasmic urge slowly fades away. After resting for a time to recuperate, Kevin resumes with easy pelvic thrusting motions.

At last, Jasmine's vagina has trapped the most personal part of Kevin's body. She can see how much she is pleasing him. Jasmine knows that she is the only one who can capture him like this, anytime she wants to. But at first, she thought that her enlarged clitoral bulbs and their strong muscles wouldn't allow Kevin's enormous organ in. And when it penetrated, Jasmine felt some pain and it wasn't imagined. Fortunately, the discomfort slowly gave way to pleasant sexual sensations.

Now, Kevin's slow back-and-forth movements begin to stretch the strong muscles of her vagina allowing more and more of his penis to enter. As their organs gradually adjust to each other, Jasmine flexes her powerful PC muscles increasing her vagina's grip on the shaft of Kevin's penis.

Jasmine feels the sexual sensations emanating up from the enlarged clitoral bulbs that are being massaged by the thrusting of Kevin's penis within her vagina. She can also feel the erogenous sensations coming from the swollen glans of her clitoris, as its hypersensitive corona is massaged by the hood that is pulled up-and-down by the tense inner lips below.

Gaining confidence, Kevin allows his pelvic tilting and thrusting movements to grow stronger and deeper. Then like playing his favorite pastime, Texas Hold 'Em poker, Kevin goes "all in." The glans of his penis finally meets the back wall of her vagina, and Kevin's organ is now a perfect fit for Jasmine.

Kevin is extremely happy because the "all in" fullness feels so awesome. It feels like he is having an out-of-body experience. But instead of telling Jasmine how wonderful he feels, he just opens his mouth and utters low moans and groans.

Regaining some control, Kevin asks Jasmine to wrap her arms around his neck. He wants to exchange places with her, to relieve some of the built-up sexual pressures and to contain his urges. With one smooth roll, Jasmine straddles above him like a racehorse jockey.

(One of Jasmine's most significant secrets is that whenever she is superior to Kevin, she naturally assumes a position of total control and is free to make her own "special" sexual massaging motions.)

Jasmine sighs in relief now that Kevin's weight and pressure have been taken off of her. But as her warm, damp back is opened to the cool air, she notices an annoying itch spreading out rapidly from her spine.

The irritating sex flush engulfs her back and upper buttocks. Jasmine asks Kevin to scratch her itch – on the sides, in the middle and down, lower down, and up again. Kevin digs his fingernails into her back and bottom for the next several moments, while he concentrates on keeping his erection. Jasmine is in one of her best lovemaking positions, and her momentum begins to build.

At this point, Kevin is just trying to hold on and to go that extra mile. He has been able to last for at least two to three times longer than the time some men take to complete the entire sex act. But Kevin continues to keep Jasmine aroused by deep kissing, as well as breast fondling, sucking, and suckling.

(Kevin has two personal secrets to holding on. First, when flat on his back, Kevin is in the best position for holding on. And second, Kevin must not tense his large gluteal buttock muscles; nor can he make any quick pelvic tilting and thrusting motions using his thigh, abs, and lower back muscles.)

Now that the itch of her sex flush has been relieved, Jasmine can focus on her orgasm. *Sustained sexual stimulation to the breasts, vulva, clitoris, and urethra is Jasmine's personal secret to attaining her orgasm, and she is well aware of this secret.*

Jasmine performs some of her special pelvic tilting and pumping undulations by alternately flexing and releasing her abs and lower back muscles. She begins to "bear down" by increasing the massaging pressures of the hypersensitive glans of her clitoris against the upper surfaces of Kevin's organ and pubic mound. Jasmine's wavelike pelvic motions also stimulate her highly sensitive urethra along the wrinkled urethral ridge. Also being excited are her swollen clitoral bulbs, as they place sexually stimulating and choking pressures on the shaft of Kevin's enclosed organ.

At first, when Jasmine's clitoris had become erect, the glans and body rose slightly outward and upward, as the glans had emerged (or had tried to emerge) from under the hood. But as her clitoral erection advanced, the contractions of the clitoral leg muscles tended to pull the glans of her clitoris back under the covering hood. Now, the hypersensitive glans of Jasmine's clitoris may be in the best position to be stimulated to her orgasm.

As her climax approaches, Jasmine exclaims, "Quick, Kevie, I can feel it coming!"

"Okay, Jazzy," Kevin replies.

"Oooh … hurry, hurry up!" She swoons.

Jasmine and Kevin are about to experience the secrets of their convulsive, out-of-this-world orgasms.

chapter

7 Secrets of the Third Phase

Jasmine and Kevin are about to experience the most deeply pleasurable and intensely gratifying sensations achieved during this phase. On one hand, Jasmine's and Kevin's orgasms might be subdued and hard to detect, yet on the other, either or both could undergo a violent convulsion!

Jasmine feels the effects of her fast-approaching orgasm as the hypo-T advances her heart rate, blood pressure, breathing rate, and body temperature. But she seems to be bothered by the tensing of random body muscles (myotonia) and the accompanying psychic conditioning signals that are building in the higher centers of her brain.

While kneeling and straddling his hips, Jasmine feels the pressure of Kevin's whole penis within her vagina. Jasmine takes great pleasure in being able to capture his entire member and shows her delight by massaging it slowly with her special rhythmic pelvic tilting and pumping undulations.

By riding back-and-forth on his organ, Jasmine applies steady massaging pressures to her vulva, the sensitive urethra along the wrinkled urethral ridge and the hypersensitive glans of her clitoris. She also feels the sexual sensations radiating up from her swollen elongated clitoral bulbs as they pick up the thrusting of Kevin's penis within her vagina.

It appears that Jasmine is definitely following her secret keys of sustained sexual stimulation that will lead the way to her orgasm.

With Jasmine supported by her shins and knees, she draws back and upward causing her vagina to pull on the shaft of Kevin's penis. Then she scoots down and forward engulfing it, as she stretches down and plants a full, wet kiss right on his surprised lips.

Jasmine's rhythmic pelvic tilting and pumping undulations continue to grow stronger, as her strokes get faster and deeper. She wants to increase her vagina's grip on Kevin's penis, so she flexes her potent PC muscles. The powerful PC muscle action energizes her other pelvic floor muscles to quickly tighten around Kevin's enclosed penis.

By being a passive yet occupied partner, Kevin continues to hang on, as his organ is still in the solid, rigid erection phase. Kevin tries to keep himself stable but is being excited by the sight of Jasmine's breasts jiggling in front of him.

Kevin continues to arouse Jasmine by fondling her firm breasts and rolling her erect nipples between his fingers. From time to time, he stops her actions to suck and suckle one tense nipple, and then the other.

Again, the unexpected secret is that Kevin's suckling is prompting Jasmine's hypo-T to release more oxytocin into her bloodstream.

Since Jasmine is certainly not pregnant, the hormone continues to squeezes out only a scant amount of fluid from her mammary glands. Oxytocin also increases the contractions of her uterus and causes it to rise.

Perhaps Kevin has been able to hang on because Jasmine has been careful not to overly stimulate the glans of his penis. Fortunately, her "all in" and back-and-forth massaging motions were focused at the base of his organ. If Jasmine had pulled back and made shallow in-and-out movements, this action would have placed extreme skin friction and deep pressures on Kevin's thin-skinned glans and its highly sensitive corona.

Also, in the past few moments, Kevin noticed that Jasmine's sexual massaging motions were intensifying, growing tighter and more frantic. As Kevin continues to enjoy Jasmine's sensational activity, he soaks in every stroke, squeeze, rub, or tug. But Kevin knows that he has to keep holding on for just a little longer.

Her breathing is rapid, as Jasmine tries to keep up with her racing heart. Her fever rises, causing her body to perspire. Everywhere, random body muscles are tensing and relaxing, all by themselves.

Since her legs have been bent for quite some time, Jasmine wants to stretch them out. While leaning on Kevin's chest and pointing with her toes, she straightens both legs in one quick motion. Jasmine is now surfing straight on his abdomen, but her legs still straddle Kevin's thighs, as the weight of her lower body puts increasing pressures on his organ.

Feeling the urge, Jasmine flexes her large gluteal buttock muscles that automatically pull the inside thigh muscles causing her legs to close. As her buttocks come together, Kevin's penis is clamped in her two-legged vise.

"Oh, yes!" Kevin says. But instead, he might say, "Oh, no, not again," as he feels the surging fullness of emission and then the explosive ejaculation!

Kevin was just trying his best to keep steady, but Jasmine's moves were too quick and intense for him to handle.

Shortly, Kevin hears Jasmine's three lonely words, "What about me?"

(Because of the intensity of their sexplay or his normal reaction timing, Kevin could climax at any time. But if he is able to take the added pressures after Jasmine's quick moves, Kevin will get yet another chance, and the orgasm phase continues.)

While surfing on his abdomen, Jasmine smiles slyly when she hears Kevin's low groan from the choking of his trapped organ. She tries to make some up-and-down and side-to-side wiggling motions like a fish struggling on dry land, but these movements take too much effort, so she stops.

Jasmine notices that Kevin's penis has slipped out from its "all in" position, and she has lost the "feeling of fullness" that she relishes. Raising her upper body with her arms, Jasmine decides to return to the riding position. Opening her legs, Jasmine slides her knees up and around Kevin's hips and is riding "all in" again.

It's been quite some time since Kevin began holding on, and Jasmine has been doing all the "work." He was anxious and thought that it was all over, especially when Jasmine straightened her legs and closed them in on his organ. For a moment, he felt his penis slipping out, but fortunately, she moved "all in" again. Overall, Kevin is satisfied and perhaps her orgasm is now only a few heartbeats away.

Knowing that Kevin is waiting for her, Jasmine is doing everything possible to speed up her secret keys of sustained sexual stimulation.

Jasmine is keenly aware of her approaching orgasm. Her radiating clitoris continues to send increasing sexual sensations to her higher cerebral centers and hypo-T. Jasmine also notices the other signs of her rapidly approaching orgasm.

Her swollen nipples ache, so Jasmine cups her favored breast and offers it to him. Kevin sucks and suckles it, and then the other, as Jasmine's hypo-T releases more oxytocin into her bloodstream.

The stimulating hormone continues to support the rising and swelling of Jasmine's breasts. Oxytocin also causes the uterus to contract and elevate into a "tenting" position, enlarging the inner two-thirds of her vagina and making it deeper.

While Kevin is trying to remain steady, Jasmine slides both of her clammy hands on his hands and intertwines her fingers with his. Straightening both arms, she pins him down with all her might!

Bracing on her hands, Jasmine slowly raises her head and arches her back, as the weight of her upper body slides directly down her spine. This focuses the pressures of her urethra, clitoris, vulva, and vagina directly onto the shaft of Kevin's enclosed organ.

Wanting to increase her vagina's grip on Kevin's penis, Jasmine rhythmically flexes her powerful PC muscles. The contractions automatically energize her vaginal and other pelvic floor muscles to tighten around his enclosed organ.

Riding "all in," Jasmine can't press forward, so she quickly draws back and upward using her abs, lower back, and thigh muscles. She then slides her pelvis forward to the "all-in" position. Jasmine keeps repeating this cycle, pumping backwards-and-forwards, in-and-out, as her sexual motions continue to build in strength and quickness.

Jasmine releases Kevin's hands so that he can help with her special pelvic tilting and pumping undulations. While holding her hips, Kevin can guide her away and by grasping her buttocks, he can draw her back up against him.

Suddenly, Jasmine drops her head downward and swings her upper torso to her right. She then forces her right knee in-between his legs and makes a sliding move with her pelvis up toward his organ, and she rides "all in" again.

Her legs straddle his right thigh, as both bodies form a sort of open scissors or an X. Jasmine pulls her arms around Kevin's neck and gives him a deep kiss. Continuing with her rhythmic pelvic tilting and pumping undulations, Jasmine feels the mounting muscle tensions and sexual sensations.

Jasmine's higher cerebral centers and hypo-T continue to escalate her vital signs. Her normal heart rate of 72 beats per minute is now racing somewhere up to 180 beats or more. Trying to keep up with her pounding heart, Jasmine gasps for air and might unknowingly be hyperventilating. Minute beads of sweat glisten on her neck, chest, abdomen, and elsewhere on her sweltering body.

Random muscles from all over her body are rapidly twitching in spasms that are intense and irritable because Jasmine can't control them. Her feet might start unusual, intense flexing (carpopedal spasms), as all of her toes flex wide apart or the big toe cramps upward and the rest of her toes curl under.

As the buildup of her fast-approaching orgasm heightens, Jasmine tightens her pelvic floor and powerful PC muscles, the anal sphincter muscles, the other muscles surrounding the vagina, and the strong muscles of the elongated clitoral bulbs.

These are the muscles that are instantly activated during a healthy sneeze, a deep cough, or an oncoming orgasm. The same muscles also make-up the "Indian death grip" that her vagina has on Kevin's penis. Jasmine has a powerful sensation of bearing down, as though she is about to push Kevin's organ out of her vagina.

Jasmine is extremely aware of the mounting psychic and physical sexual sensations that are being sent to her higher cerebral centers and hypo-T. At the same time, Jasmine can feel her body expanding and tightening like a balloon that is getting ready to explode. Still straddling Kevin's right thigh, Jasmine tenses her abdominal muscles, as the special undulating movements of her pelvis continue to increase in intensity and speed.

The rhythmic pumping motions place intense pressures on the sensitive urethra along the wrinkled urethral ridge and on the hypersensitive glans and swollen bulbs of her clitoris. Jasmine's secret keys of sustained sexual stimulation have brought her to the apex of her climax.

Gradually, Jasmine's face grimaces, as if she's really angry. While bracing on her hands again, she closes her eyes and clenches her fists with all her might. As her neck muscles tighten, she slowly bows her head down. Jasmine wants to scream, but all she can muster is a high-pitched whimper in a dry parched throat as she jerks her head up!

"I'm coming!" Jasmine exclaims.

The massive buildup of psychic and physical sexual tensions reaches its peak and is suddenly released, as Jasmine begins to experience her orgasm.

She initially might see (in her mind's eye) the flash of a blinding white light or perhaps some exploding multi-colored stars. Jasmine could feel like falling or even lifting and floating away.

Her whole lower body quivers, as Jasmine feels the involuntary contractions of the anal sphincter muscles, the clitoral leg muscles, the powerful PC muscles, the four other vaginal muscles, and the ringed muscle encircling her urethra and vagina.

The initial three to six contractions pulsate at varied rates of about one to three per second. Nearing the end of the initial muscle tensing, Jasmine feels the orgasmic reflex, the equally rapid four to six intense spasms of the strong muscles of her elongated clitoral bulbs. The muscle tightening and releasing continues onward at slower pulses and fading strength as Jasmine slowly exhales a sigh of relief and fulfillment.

In future encounters, Jasmine could have a "minor" orgasm, one that is nice, tingly, pleasant, or affectionately satisfying. Now, however, she has this extremely intense orgasm, leading to a feeling of total physical release and psychic gratification. Jasmine is deeply aware of the growing sense of warmth that is emanating from the lower center of her abdomen, rising up to the level of her lungs, and flowing downward into her legs.

Meanwhile, before Jasmine's orgasm, Kevin is trying his best to hold on. Since Jasmine is "all in," her vaginal contractions are focused mainly at the base of his organ. Fortunately, not much pressure is being applied to his penile glans and its highly sensitive corona.

It appears that Kevin is maintaining his personal secrets to holding on. He is not flexing the large gluteal muscles in his buttocks, nor is he making any pelvic tilting and thrusting motions with his thighs, abs, or lower back muscles. He is also not tightening any of the pelvic floor muscles. Kevin is just trying to keep himself and his erection steady.

As Jasmine's sexual tensions build, Kevin feels a rough patch of skin (sex flush) on the upper half of her buttocks. The goose bumps may also appear on the opposite side of Jasmine's body, on her lower abdomen, in the area that is usually covered by a teeny-weeny bikini.

The noteworthy secret about the sex flush is that the gooseflesh achieves its greatest roughness and widest distribution just before the moment of Jasmine's orgasm. But Kevin might not be aware of this secret.

Jasmine's rhythmic pelvic tilting and pumping undulations become faster and stronger, shorter and more frantic, until she makes her final "all in" move. As her orgasm begins, all of the pelvic floor muscles surrounding her vagina begin their involuntary pulsating contractions.

Then, Kevin feels Jasmine's orgasmic reflex – the strong, rapid tensing of her clitoral bulb muscles that tighten and release rhythmically around the walls of her vagina and his enclosed penis. Another of his personal secrets is that this is how Kevin knows when Jasmine has climaxed.

Amazingly, Kevin has managed to keep himself steady for a long time and realizes that it is time for his orgasm. He wants to go back to the starting position so that Jasmine can rest. Quickly, Kevin gives her a bear hug and, in one easy roll, he is in position above her.

Kevin knows that because Jasmine could have another orgasm within a period of time, he can continue to make thrusting motions without any loss of skin friction on his organ. If he needs more pressure, he can ask Jasmine to tighten her pelvic floor muscles, especially the powerful PC muscles.

He could also pull back toward Jasmine's lower vagina and the strong muscles of her elongated clitoral bulbs. While making shallow thrusting motions, he can place deep pressures and skin friction on his thin-skinned glans and its highly sensitive corona. If the approaching climactic sensations become too intense, Kevin could always move "all in" and rest. He then might resume by making extremely deep thrusting motions.

Kevin could even try other positions with Jasmine's cooperation. Without her help, he won't have many options. But Kevin might still vary the position of her legs so that they are over his shoulders, straight out, or around his waist. He can also bend Jasmine's knees up to her breasts.

With his orgasm quickly approaching, Kevin feels the intense throbbing coming from the thin-skinned glans and the bulging urethra as his penis glides smoothly back-and-forth in Jasmine's vagina. This is Kevin's personal secret for thrusting to attain his orgasm.

While thrusting, Kevin tightens the muscles of the urethra, the two cylinder legs, the anal sphincter, the powerful PC, the pelvic floor, and the bulb of his penis. These are the same muscles that Kevin commonly uses to control the flow of urine or to squeeze the final drops out of his urethra. Tensing these muscles, Kevin continues to make pelvic tilting and thrusting motions that build in strength, length, and speed.

After sensing the overpowering buildup of sexual sensations and psychic conditioning signals in his higher cerebral centers and hypo-T, Kevin quickly thrusts his pelvis forward in his deepest "all in" move.

Kevin immediately feels the surging fullness of emission and then the jolting psychic release. It begins by Kevin seeing (in his mind's eye) a great flash of blinding white light that is more like a lightning bolt than a quick camera flash. Or he might see the colorful blast of exploding stars, like the kind seen after a knockout blow to the head or drawn in comic books.

In the midst of the psychic effects, Kevin's whole lower body shudders as the muscles of the urethra, the two cylinder leg muscles, the anal sphincter muscles, the potent PC muscles, and the strong muscles of the bulb of the penis begin their powerful involuntary flexing.

The initial compressions pulsate at the rate of about one to two per second, as semen containing 300 million sperm (Kevin's average) forcefully spurts out of his urethra. He experiences an incredible feeling of sexual pleasure as the semen gushes out. The pulsating muscle tensing begins to slow down, but grows more and more intense, until Kevin becomes very still.

The explosive "high" of his orgasm creates a great psychic and physical sensation that is difficult to put into words. Surely, every sexual episode may not be as spectacular as this one. But every climactic release brings him incredible gratification. This is why Kevin will always look forward to sexual encounters with Jasmine.

Kevin has been able to last an amazingly long time. From erection to psychic events, to emission and ejaculation, these events make up his climax. Kevin has very little control over most of them because the involuntary actions are controlled by his higher cerebral centers, hypo-T and spinal cord. Once activated, the climactic events are automatic, almost exactly like Jasmine's orgasm.

A few moments later, Kevin hears Jasmine's three lovely words, "Did you come?"

"Yes, Jazzy, I came," Kevin replies.

(As Kevin lies on his back, the profound "one flesh" vanishes, and two people suddenly reappear.)

What about the simultaneous orgasm? Because an orgasm is triggered by the higher cerebral centers, hypo-T, and spinal cord, it may be impossible for Kevin or Jasmine to coordinate the timing of their involuntarily controlled orgasms to occur at the same instant.

The miraculous secret, however, is that once in a great while, a simultaneous orgasm could come about by accident, magnificent timing, or remarkably good luck. (Good luck!)

Jasmine says, "Ke-evie, I'm so proud of you, waiting for me like that. Now I know why I love you so much! And, oooh, I think that was the most magnificent, breathtaking, mind and body rapture ever! My head was spinning, I felt like I was falling, and I ... I just lost it!"

"And wow, Jazzy, your orgasmic reflex was awesome!" Kevin replies.

"The next time, Kevie, I want to come again and again and again!" Jasmine goes on.

"Okay, Honey," Kevin replies. "Let's go to the next chapter. It's about the afterglow, you know – afterplay!"

8 Secrets of the Fourth Phase

Addictive Afterplay

As Kevin relaxes, the hypo-T begins to normalize his elevated heart and breathing rates, and blood pressure. His body begins to cool and enters a time of recovery called the refractory period.

The final phase is usually characterized by Kevin's reduced sensitivity to sexual arousal and inability to initiate another sexual episode. Fortunately, when Kevin is young, the refractory period might be measured in a matter of minutes. When he's older, however, the minutes could turn into hours or, alas, even days.

At times, Kevin might decide to go for another orgasm, so he continues with thrusting movements in Jasmine's vagina. But instead of experiencing positive sensations of pleasure, he suffers pain.

The mysterious afterplay secret is that this happens because the PNS nerve signals that were maintaining his erection have been overcome by the SNS nerve signals that are deflating his penis and drawing his body into the recovery period.

65

Although he is hurting, Kevin continues thrusting. But as the moments go by, instead of relenting, the pain continues to grow until it becomes so excruciating that he has to stop.

The unpredictable afterplay secret is that if Kevin is able to break through the suffering and the PNS nerve signals are restored, another sexual session would then be possible.

As Jasmine relaxes, the hypo-T begins to lower her high heart and breathing rates, and blood pressure. Her body begins to cool, and the relaxation of the walls of her vagina allows the uterus to return to its normal resting position.

The organs containing erectile tissues, such as the inner lips, clitoris, urethra, and vagina, are the slowest to normalize and may remain uncomfortably congested with blood after the end of sexual activities.

The marvelous afterplay secret is that because her body does not enter a refractory period like Kevin, Jasmine can experience another orgasm.

Because an orgasm frees the massive buildup of sexual tension, the sudden release could act like a powerful knockout. On rare occasions, Jasmine or Kevin could momentarily lose consciousness as either might experience a phenomenon the French call "petit mort," or "little death." But more often, the climactic release simply eases them to sleep.

After their mutual orgasms, Jasmine and Kevin drift along in a peaceful state of natural weariness. They soak in feelings of quiet peacefulness, profound physical gratification, and whole-body satisfaction.

As their bodies return to the unexcited state, their minds slowly reawaken, and their senses gradually regain full acuity. This afterglow time of calm and restful alertness is called afterplay.

There are four more remarkable secrets about the afterglow. First, afterplay could secretly help a marriage and may be the most important time during the sexual episode.

But because of fatigue, many couples simply doze off. Often, the afterglow is omitted. Kevin and Jasmine are urged to make full use of this time, not to start playing again, but to communicate!

Second, afterglow may secretly be the best time to say those three awesome words, "I love you." Afterplay may also be a good time to humbly say, "I'm sorry." This is because it may support saying life's three most difficult words, "I forgive you." It may also be the perfect time to quietly settle a recent problem.

The afterglow may be a good time to apologize for forgetting to take out the trash, or for teasing her cat or his dog. It might be the best time for Kevin to get permission to buy that classic sports car, or for Jasmine to shop for her new diamond ring.

Third, the best "peace talks" and good, long, friendly conversations could secretly take place during afterplay.

The promoters are the human body's own opioids, opiate-like substances (endorphins, enkephalins, and dynorphins) that are released by the hypo-T and other areas of the brain. Jasmine's and Kevin's natural painkillers and mind enhancers are the reasons for the feeling of effortless well-being and tranquility that are experienced after their orgasms.

The "natural" opioids can fit into and trigger every one of the pleasure-producing and pain-canceling nerve centers that opiates such as heroin, opium, or concentrated morphine would. The resulting euphoric high appears to be the "great peacemaker" and could explain why Jasmine and Kevin may soon be – "addicted to love."

During afterplay, Jasmine and Kevin should try to keep connected by touching, holding hands, playful kissing, cuddling, or hugging.

The fourth secret is that they should continue to talk and above all, stay awake!

Who went to the bathroom, or was it to get a snack? Are Jasmine and Kevin paying attention, or did someone suddenly fall temporarily unconscious? Who knows, if the friendly talk continues long enough and his body recuperates, Kevin will be ready for another sexual session.

But Jasmine quickly says:
- ❖ *"Oh no, Kevin, not again!"*
- ❖ *"Please, make it go away!"*
- ❖ *"I came already."*
- ❖ *"Love you!"*
- ❖ *"Zzzzzzzz."*

But Kevin muddles, "Hmmm, I wonder why I can't I stay awake? Ah, maybe it's those natural opioids or could it be those endogenous morphines that knock me out?"

"Maybe you've been working too hard, Kevie, but I still love you very much," Jasmine says.

"By the way, Jazzy, I'm sorry, but I forgot to put the toilet seat back down," he confesses.

"Don't worry, Kev, I'm always very careful – about that," she replies.

"Thanks, Honey," Kevin says. "Come on, Jazzy, let's leave with some parting words on all the secrets we've found in my father's book."

chapter

9 Secrets of the Conclusion

The End of the Beginning

These are the secrets of how marital sex mysteriously merges Jasmine and Kevin into one – two spirits believing as one, two minds trusting as one, two hearts beating as one, and two lives loving as one, as the One who created them intended.

Jasmine kept herself for Kevin and he saved himself for her because sex in a marriage is pure, holy, and free from guilt. It is a binding force that is worthy of reverence and respect. Marital sex leads to spiritual blessings and, when blessed, a family.

Always remember that the sex act superbly satisfies the unique spiritual, mental, and physical needs of a married couple. Whether Kevin and Jasmine like it more supercool than sizzling hot, more playful than really serious, more tender than erotically lustful, more kinky than strictly straight, or more "wham-bam, thank you ma'am" than slow and sweet, then that is exactly what sex is for that couple.

71

Be grateful, enjoy, and cherish the good times of sex in your marriage while patiently toughing out the rough times. Constantly build on the warm esteem, love, and intimacy, born each day of your lifelong marriage.

Always remember these closing secrets:

Compromising marital sex should give and take.

Quite often, Kevin gives love to get sex, while Jasmine gives sex to get love.

Courteous marital sex means being very patient.

Naturally, Kevin must be a gentleman, in more ways than one.

Informed marital sex is more than good luck.

When Kevin is in bed with Jasmine and doesn't know what to do, he is certainly going to need more than good luck.

Intimate marital sex means no more fears.

Jasmine and Kevin must forget about the fears of losing their individuality, impulses, and control.

Loving marital sex requires intimacy.

Kevin's and Jasmine's love for each other cannot blossom without intimacy.

Patient marital sex always requires consideration, compromise, and flexibility.

Every sexual session does not always come out just right. That's why it's so nice to try again – real soon.

Perfect marital sex requires practice.

Kevin and Jasmine must always practice and practice and practice, because good practice makes perfect.

Quality marital sex begins between your two ears.

Jasmine and Kevin always have to improve what happens in bed by learning how to do it – better.

Satisfying marital sex always answers each other's needs.

Jasmine must be in the emotional mood for love. Kevin, of course, is always in the mood.

Spontaneous marital sex means variety.

Kevin and Jasmine must learn to be creative in and, especially, out of bed.

Successful marital sex requires not only mutual love but also care and respect.

The quality of Jasmine's and Kevin's relationship and sexual function depends upon mutual love, care, and respect, or "When we're okay, I'm okay."

Thoughtful marital sex means being prepared.

It's always nice to have them on hand and ready for use.

And the final secret is:

Everlasting marital sex describes Jasmine as a great wife and lover, who can be satisfied by satisfying her husband – all his life long, and Kevin, as a great lover and husband, who can be satisfied by satisfying his wife – all her life long!

CHAPTER REFERENCES

CHAPTER 1. THE ORGANS OF ORGASM

1. Agur, Anne M.R. & Dalley II, Arthur R.,
   Grant's Atlas of Anatomy. 11th ed., Baltimore, MD;
   Lippincott, Williams & Wilkins, 2005,
   Overview of the perineum: pp. 242-243;
   Male perineum: pp. 244-255;
   Female perineum: pp. 256-263.
2. Gardner, Ernest, Gray, Donald J., O'Rahilly, Ronan, *Anatomy*.
   3rd ed., Philadelphia, PA; W.B. Saunders, 1969,
   Perineal region and external genital organs
   (male and female): pp. 511-522.
3. Goss, Charles Mayo, editor, Gray, Henry,
   Gray's Anatomy, Anatomy of the Human Body by Henry Gray.
   29th American Edition, Philadelphia, PA;
   Lea & Febinger, 1973,
   Clitoris: pp. 1331-1332;
   Penis: pp. 1310-1315.
4. Hashmat, Azid I. & Das, Sakti, editors,
   The Penis. Malvern, PA; Lea & Febiger, 1993,
   Anatomy of the penis: pp. 12-16.
5. Larsen, P. Reed, *Williams Textbook of Endocrinology*.
   10th ed., Philadelphia, PA; Saunders – An imprint of
   Elsiever Science, 2003,
   Reproduction: pp. 587-793.
6. Lowrey, Thomas P. & Thea S.,
   The Clitoris. St. Louis, MO; Warren H. Green, Inc., 1976,
   Anatomy of the human clitoris: pp. 9-75.
7. Rugh, Roberts & Shettles, Landrum B.,
   From Conception to Birth. New York, NY;
   Harper & Row, Publishers, Inc., 1971,
   The 1st and 2nd month of life, the embryo becomes the
   fetus and the third trimester: pp. 17-84.

8. Walsh, Patrick C., Editor-in-chief,
   Campbell's Urology. 8th ed., Philadelphia, PA;
   Saunders an imprint of Elsiever Science, 2002,
   Male reproductive physiology: pp. 1437-1474;
   Female sexual anatomy and physiology: pp. 1710-1733.

CHAPTER 2. THE THREE V's

1. Agur, Anne M.R. & Dalley II, Arthur R.,
   Grant's Atlas of Anatomy. 11th ed., Baltimore, MD;
   Lippincott, William & Wilkin, 2005,
   Overview of female pelvis, uterus, ovaries, and
   vagina: pp. 224-233;
   Overview of perineum: pp. 242-243;
   Overview of male perineum: pp. 244-255;
   Overview of female perineum: pp. 256-263.
2. Copeland, Larry J., *Textbook of Gynecology*.
   2nd ed., Philadelphia, PA; W.B. Saunders Co., 2000,
   Clinical anatomy of the pelvis: pp. 17-24.
3. Jones Jr., Howard W. & Jones, Georgeanna S.,
   Novak's Textbook of Gynecology. 10th ed.,
   Baltimore, MD; The Williams & Wilkins Co., 1981,
   Anatomy: pp. 1-16.
4. Moore, Keith L. & Dalley II, Arthur F.,
   Clinically Oriented Anatomy. Baltimore, MD;
   Lippincott, Williams & Wilkins, 1999,
   Female internal genital organs: vagina: pp. 370-373;
   Perineal fascia: pp. 392-395.
5. Ridley, Constance R., *The Vulva*. Philadelphia, PA;
   W.B. Saunders Co., Ltd., 1975,
   Anatomy of the vulva area: pp. 25-38.

CHAPTER 3. THE THREE E's

1. Barr, Murray L. & Kiernan, John A.,
   The Human Nervous System. 6th ed., Philadelphia, PA;
   J.B. Lippincott Co., 1993,
   Diencephalon: pp. 181-209.
2. Boron, Walter F., *Medical Physiology*. Updated ed.,
   Philadelphia, PA; Elsevier, Inc., 2005,
   Organization of the nervous system;
   Diencephalon: pp. 273-274;
   The male reproduction system; male sex act: pp.1136-1140.
3. Carson III, Culley C., Kirby, Roger S., Goldstein, Irwin,
   editors, *Textbook of Erectile Dysfunction*,
   Oxford, UK; Isis Medical Media, Ltd., 1999;
   Shetty S.D. & Farah, R.N., Anatomy of erectile
   function: pp. 25-41.
   Hendry, W.F., Causes and treatment of ejaculatory
   disorders: pp. 569-581;
   Iribarren, I. Moncada & Saenz de Tejada, I., Vascular
   physiology of penile erection: pp. 51-57;
   Chuang, A.T. & Steers, W.D., Neurophysiology of
   penile erection: pp. 59-72;
   Marson, L., Central nervous system control: pp. 73-88;
   Moreland, R.B. & Nehra, A., Pathophysiology of erectile
   dysfunction: a molecular basis, role of NPT in maintaining
   potency: pp. 105-115;
   Seftel, A.D. & Althof, S.E., Premature ejaculation:
   pp.583-587.
4. Dement, William C. & Vaughn, Christopher,
   The Promise of Sleep. New York, NY; Delacore Press Random
   House, Inc., 1999,
   A short and personal history of sleep research: pp. 27-50;
   The real life of dreams (REM sleep and NPT): pp. 290-309.
5. Fowler, Clare J., editor, *Neurology of Bladder, Bowel, and Sexual
   Dysfunction*. Woburn, MA; Butterworth-Heinemann, a
   member of the Reed Elsevier group, 1999,
   Physiology of male sexual function: pp. 47-55.

6. Ganten, Detley & Pfaff, Donald, *Sleep,Clinical and Experiment Aspects*, Berlin; Heidelberg; New York; Springer-Verlag, 1982,
Neurobiology of REM sleep by Gunter Stock: pp. 1-26.

7. Larsen, P. Reed, *Williams Textbook of Endocrinology.* 10th ed., Philadelphia, PA; Saunders an imprint of Elsiever Science, 2003,
Hypothalamus and pituitary: pp. 81-329.

8. Moore, Keith L. & Dalley II, Arthur F., *Clinically Oriented Anatomy.* Baltimore, MD; Lippincott, Williams & Wilkins, 1999,
Structures in the deep perineal pouch: pp. 396-399;
Male perineum, urethra: pp. 403-404.

9. Newman, Alfred J., *Beyond Viagra, Plain talk about treating male and female dysfunction.* Montgomery, AL; Starrhill Press, 1999,
Understanding male sexual function: pp. 9-20.

10. Walsh, Patrick C., Editor-in-chief, *Campbell's Urology.* 8th ed., Philadelphia, PA; Saunders-an imprint of Elsiever Science, 2002,
Physiology of penile erection and pathophysiology of erectile dysfunction and priapism by Tom F. Lue: pp. 1591-1618;
Male Reproductive Physiology by Peter N. Schlegel and Matthew Hardy: pp. 1437-1440.

CHAPTER 4. SEX DRIVE

1. Carson III, Culley C., Kirby, Roger S., Goldstein, Irwin, editors, *Textbook of Erectile Dysfunction.* Oxford, UK; Isis Medical Media, Ltd., 1999;
Erectile dysfunction: endocrinological therapies, risks, and benefits of treatment (androgens): pp. 327-344.

2. Rhodes, Rodney A. and Tanner, George A., editors, *Medical Physiology.* First ed., New York, NY; Little, Brown and Co., 1995;
Oogonia begin developing during fetal life: pp. 763-764.

3. Walsh, Patrick C., Editor-in-chief,
   Campbell's Urology. 8th ed., Philadelphia, PA;
   Saunders-an imprint of Elsiever Science, 2002,
   Male Sexual Function: pp. 1589-1619;
   Female sexual function: pp. 1710-1717.

CHAPTER 5. FOREPLAY

1. Botting, Kate & Douglas, *Sex Appeal, the Art and Science
   of Sexual Attraction.* London, UK; Box Tree, Ltd.,
   Broadway House, 1995,
   Brief encounter, body language from first sight to
   first sex: pp. 115-121;
   The scented ape, from scent to the pheromone factor:
   pp. 147-163.
2. Haas & Hass, Adelaide, Kurt, *Understanding Sexuality.*
   2nd ed., St. Louis, MO; Times Mirror/Mosby College
   Publishing, 1990,
   Arousal: pp.114-120.

CHAPTER 6. SEXPLAY

1. Haas & Hass, Adelaide, Kurt, *Understanding Sexuality.*
   2nd ed., St. Louis, MO; Times Mirror/Mosby College
   Publishing, 1990,
   Coitus: pp. 120-121.
2. Fowler, Clare J., editor, *Neurology of Bladder, Bowel, and Sexual
   Dysfunction.* Woburn, MA; Butterworth-Heinemann,
   a member of the Reed Elsevier group, 1999,
   Physiology of female sexual function: pp. 33-46;
   Physiology of male sexual function: pp. 47-55.

CHAPTER 7. ORGASM

1. Chang, Jolan, *The Tao of Love and Sex,*
   The Ancient Chinese Way to Ecstasy.
   New York, NY; E. P. Dutton, 1977,
   Love positions: pp. 56-63.
2. Fowler, Clare J., editor, *Neurology of Bladder, Bowel, and Sexual*
   Dysfunction. Woburn, MA; Butterworth-Heinemann,
   a member of the Reed Elsevier group, 1999,
   Physiology of female sexual function: pp. 33-46;
   Physiology of male sexual function: pp. 47-55.
3. Haas & Hass, Adelaide, Kurt, *Understanding Sexuality.*
   2nd ed., St. Louis, MO; Times Mirror/Mosby College
   Publishing, 1990, Orgasm: pp. 131-140.

CHAPTER 8. AFTERPLAY

1. Haas & Hass, Adelaide, Kurt, *Understanding Sexuality.*
   2nd ed., St. Louis, MO, Times Mirror/Mosby College
   Publishing, 1990,
   Afterplay and resolution: pp.141-144.
2. Mishell, Jr., Daniel R. & Davajan, Val & Lobo, Rogerio A.
   editors, *Infertility, Contraception & Reproductive*
   Endocrinology. 3rd ed., Cambridge, MA;
   Blackwell Scientific Publications, 1991,
   Hypothalamus, opioid peptides: pp. 16-19.
3. Grilly, David M., *Drugs and Human Behavior.*
   4th ed., Boston, MA; Allyn and Bacon, 2002,
   Endorphins: pp.87-88;
   Endogenous Opioid Peptides and their receptors:
   pp. 239-241.

BIBLIOGRAPHY

1. Boron, Walter F. & Boulpaep, Emile L.,
   Medical Physiology. Updated ed., Philadelphia, PA;
   Elsevier Saunders, 2005.
2. Carson III, Culley C. & Kirby, Roger S. & Goldstein, Irwin,
   editors, *Textbook of Erectile Dysfunction*,
   Oxford, UK; Isis Medical Media, Ltd., 1999.
3. Douglas M. Anderson, MA, chief lexicographer,
   Dorland's Illustrated Medical Dictionary.
   28th ed., Philadelphia, PA; W.B. Saunders Co., 1994.
4. Germann, William J. & Stanfield, Cindy L.,
   Principles of Human Physiology, San Francisco, CA; Pearson
   Education, Inc., publishing as Benjamin Cummings, 2002.
5. Goldstein, Bernard, *Introduction to Human Sexuality*,
   New York, NY; McGraw-Hill, Inc., 1976
6. Goss, Charles Mayo, editor, Gray, Henry,
   Gray's Anatomy, Anatomy of the Human Body.
   29th ed., Philadelphia, PA; Lea & Febinger, 1973.
7. Guyton, Arthur C., *Textbook of Medical Physiology*.
   8th ed., Philadelphia, PA; W.B. Saunders Co., 1991.
8. Katchadourian, Herant A. & Lunde, Donald T.,
   Fundamentals of Human Sexuality. 2nd ed., New York, NY;
   Holt, Reinehart and Windston, 1975.
9. Kinsey, Alfred C. & Associates:
   Sexual Behavior in the Human Male, Philadelphia, PA;
   W.B. Saunders Co., 1948;
   Sexual Behavior in the Human Female, Philadelphia, PA;
   W.B. Saunders Co., 1953.
10. Krandel, Eric R. & Schwartz, James H. & Jessell, Thomas,
    Principles of Neural Science. 3rd ed., East Norwalk, CT;
    Appleton & Lange, 1991.
11. Larsen, William J.,
    Anatomy, Development Function Clinical Correlations,
    Philadelphia, PA; Elsevier Science (USA), 2002.

12. Marieb, Elaine N., *Human Anatomy and Physiology.* 2nd ed., Redwood City, CA; The Benjamin Cummings Publishing Co., Inc., 1992.

13. McCracken, Thomas O., *New Atlas of Human Anatomy,* Metro Books, an imprint of Friedman/Fairfax Publishers by arrangement with Anatographica, LLC, 2000.

14. Masters, William H. & Johnson, Virginia E., *Human Sexual Response.* 1st ed., London, UK; J. & A. Churchill, Ltd., 1966.

15. Pritchard, Jack A. & McDonald, Paul C., *Williams Obstetrics.* 15th ed., New York, NY; Appleton-Century-Crofts, A publishing division of Prentice-Hall, 1976.

16. Schover, Leslie R. & Thomas Jr., Anthony J., *Overcoming Male Infertility,* New York, NY; John Wiley & Sons, Inc., 2000.

17. Tortora, Gerard J. & Grabowski, Sandra R., *Principles of Anatomy and Physiology.* 10th ed., New York, NY; Biological Sciences Textbooks, Inc. and Sandra Grabowski, 2003.

anatomy: study of the structure of the body, and how its parts relate to one another.

androgen: any substance that promotes masculinization; masculinizing hormones produced by the testes in males and adrenal cortex in both sexes (see glands, adrenal and testosterone).

anus: distal end and outlet of the rectum.

aphrodisiac: any substance that when ingested increases sexual motivation.

areola: area surrounding the nipple of the breast.

artery: blood vessel that carries blood away from the heart.

atresia: degeneration and re-absorption of an ovarian follicle before it fully matures.

autonomic nervous system (ANS): consisting of three divisions, sympathetic, parasympathetic, and enteric that conduct nerve impulses from the CNS to smooth muscle, cardiac muscle, glands, and digestive tract. So named because this part of the nervous system was thought to be self-governing but is not so; divisions are regulated by the hypothalamus and higher cerebral centers.

biological clock: see circadian rhythm.

blood flow: amount of blood flowing through the vessel or organ at a particular time.

brain: that part of the CNS contained within the cranium, comprising the prosencephalon, mesencephalon, and rhombencephalon.

brain stem: the stalklike portion of the brain connecting the cerebral hemispheres with the spinal cord comprising the mesencephalon, pons, and medulla oblongata.

Buck's fascia: the deep fascia of the penis named after Gurdon Buck, an American surgeon.

bulbs of the vestibule: (homologues of the male penile bulb) anteriorly the bulbs meet at the junction (commissura bulborum) that by a narrow band of erectile tissue (pars intermedia) runs the length of the body before expanding into the glans clitoris; clitoral bulbs.

carpopedal spasm: muscle contractions of the hands and feet occurring during peaks of sexual tension.

central nervous system (CNS): the brain and spinal cord.

cerebellum: part of the brain lying posterior to the medulla oblongata and pons; governs balance and coordinates skilled movements.

cerebral cortex: surface of the cerebral hemispheres consisting of gray matter; processes information relating to the senses, thought, memory, and movement.

cerebrum: two hemispheres of the forebrain; largest part of the brain; involved in conscious thought, feelings, and movement.

cervix: mouth-like part of the uterus that opens into the vagina.

chromosome: one of the small threadlike structures in the nucleus of a cell, normally 46 in a human diploid cell that bears the genetic material; composed of DNA and proteins; contain genes, the instructions needed to construct and run the body.

circadian rhythm: cycle of active and nonactive periods in organisms determined by internal mechanisms and repeating about every 24 hours; may also be called the biological clock.

climax: peak period or moments of greatest sexual intensity; orgasm.

clitoral bulbs: see bulbs of the vestibule.

clitoris: female genital tubercle homologous to the male penis; an erectile organ similar in structure and function to the male penis, except for urination; consists of the glans, body, legs, and bulbs.

commissura bulborum: commissure: a site of union of corresponding parts; in the clitoris, the junction of the clitoral bulbs (bulbs of the vestibule) and pars intermedia.

conception: union of the ovum and sperm that forms a visible zygote.

contraction: to shorten or develop tension, an ability highly developed in muscle cells.

corona: crown-like eminence or encircling structure; the rounded proximal border of the glans, separated from the corpora cavernosa of the penis or clitoris.

corpus callosum: arched mass of white matter, composed primarily of transverse fibers connecting the left and right cerebral hemispheres.

corpus cavernosum: cavernous body or spongy body; a column of erectile tissue forming the dorsum and sides of the clitoris or penis; plural, corpora cavernosa.

corpus spongiosum penis: column of erectile tissue that forms the urethral surface of the penis and in which the urethra is found; its distal expansion forms the glans penis.

crus: tapered portion of corpus cavernosum; leg; crura, plural.

diencephalon: part of forebrain; between cerebral hemispheres and midbrain; includes the thalamus, hypothalamus, epithalamus, and subthalamus; may be considered part of the brain stem; called also *interbrain.*

dorsal: pertaining to the back; posterior.

ductus (vas) deferens: duct that carries sperm from the epididymus to ampulla and the excretory duct of the seminal vesicle to form the ejaculatory duct; a.k.a., spermatic cord, seminal duct.

dynorphins: may be involved with pain regulation at the levels of the spinal cord and medulla and may aid hypothalamic regulation of eating and drinking; see also opioid, endorphin, and enkephalin.

ejaculation: ejection or expulsion of semen from the penis during orgasm; reflex or involuntary response to a stimulus.

ejaculation center: nerves that emanate from the thoracic and lumbar vertebrae of the spinal cord.

ejaculatory duct: canal formed by the union of the ductus deferens and the excretory duct of the seminal vesicle that enters the prostatic part of the urethra.

embryo: name of unborn child during the first eight weeks of development after fertilization.

emission: propulsion of sperm into the urethra due to peristaltic contractions of the ducts of the testes, epididymides, seminal vesicles, and ductus (vas) deferens from sympathetic neuron stimulation.

endocrine system: body system that includes internal organs that secrete hormones.

endorphin: neuropeptide in the central nervous system; acts as a painkiller – more potent than morphine; see also opioid, dynorphin, and enkephalin.

enkephalin: functions as neurotransmitter at many locations in the brain and spinal cord and plays a part in pain perception, movement, mood, behavior, and neuroendocrine regulation; see also opioid, dynorphin, and endorphin.

epididymus: comma-shaped organ attached to testis; containing the ductus epididymus, in which sperm undergo maturation; plural, epididymides.

epithelium: covering of internal and external surfaces of the body, including the lining of vessels and other small cavities.

erectile dysfunction: abnormality of clitoral or penile erectile function.

erection: enlarged and stiff state of the clitoris or penis resulting from the engorgement of the spongy erectile tissue with blood.

erection center: comprised of nerves emanating from three vertebrae of the sacrum, S2 to S4.

estrogen: feminizing hormones synthesized by the ovaries; govern development of oocytes, maintenance of female reproductive structures, and appearance of secondary sex characteristics; also affect fluid and electrolyte balance, and protein anabolism; the most potent of which is estradiol; others are estrone and estriol.

external anal sphincters: constricts the anus.

fallopian tube: see also uterine tube.

fascia: fibrous membrane; covers, supports, and separates muscles.

fetus: developing human from the ninth week to birth.

fibromembranous: composed of membrane containing fibrous tissue.

fibromuscular: composed of fibrous and muscular tissue.

fibrosis: formation of fibrous tissue.

flaccid: relaxed, flabby or soft; lacking muscle tone.

follicle: small secretory sac or cavity; group of cells that contains a developing oocyte in the ovaries.

follicle-stimulating hormone (FSH): hypothalamus-regulated production of FSH by the anterior pituitary, initiates the development of ova, and stimulates ovaries to secrete estrogens in females and initiates sperm production in the testes in males.

frenulum: small fold of mucus membrane that connects two parts and limits movement; the union of the two medial parts of the labia minora in the female and the lower fold of the prepuce in the male.

gamete: male or female reproductive cell; sperm cell or secondary oocyte.

gene: biological unit of heredity; a segment of DNA located in a definite position on a particular chromosome.

genital tubercle: that part of the genitalia that develops into the free body and glans of the clitoris or penis.

gland: specialized epithelial cell or cells that secrete substances; may be exocrine or endocrine.

gland, adrenal: situated at the cranial pole of each kidney, one of two flattened bodies that comprises two components: cortex under control of the pituitary elaborates steroid hormones and medulla elaborates the catecholamines epinephrine and norephinephrine.

gland, Bartholin's: one of two small mucus bodies situated under and behind the clitoral bulb that secretes mucus into a groove at the hymenal ridge; homologue of the male bulbourethral or Cowper's gland; a.k.a., gland, greater vestibular.

gland, Cowper's: situated within the urogenital diaphragm, one of two pea-shaped glands that secretes a clear, alkaline fluid into the cavernous urethra neutralizing the urethra; a.k.a., gland, bulbourethral.

gland, endocrine: ductless gland that empties its hormonal products directly into the blood.

gland, exocrine: gland that secretes its products into ducts that carry the secretions into body cavities into the lumen of an organ, or to the outer surface of the body.

gland, greater vestibular: gland, paired, on either side of the vaginal introitus that by ducts open outside of the hymenal ridge; see also gland, Bartholin's.

glands, mammary: modified sudoriferous (sweat) glands of the female breasts that produce milk for nourishment of the young.

gland, prostate: doughnut-shaped gland inferior to the urinary bladder that surrounds the superior portion of the male urethra and secretes a seminal fluid containing acid phosphatase, citric acid and proteolytic enzymes, which causes liquefaction of coagulated semen.

gland, Skene's: group of para-urethral glands of the female urethra named after American gynecologist Alexander Skene.

gland, thymus: the site of production and storage of T lymphocytes (T cells of the immune system); consists of two pyramidal lobes.

gland, thyroid: one of the two endocrine glands that secretes hormones regulating the body's metabolic rate.

glycogen: highly branched polymer of glucose containing thousands of subunits; functions as a compact store of glucose molecules in liver and muscle fibers (cells).

gonad: gland that produces gametes and hormones; testis or ovary.

gray matter: areas in the central nervous system and ganglia containing neuronal cell bodies, dendrites, unmyelinated axons, axon terminals, and neuroglia. Nissl bodies impart a gray color and there is little or no myelin in gray matter.

heart: hollow muscular organ lying slightly to the left of the midline of the chest that pumps the blood through the cardiovascular system.

homeostasis: condition in which the body's internal environment remains relatively constant, within physiological limits.

homologous: parts or organs corresponding in structure but not necessarily in function.

hormone: secretion of endocrine cells that alters the physiological activity of target cells in the body.

hymen: thin fold of vascularized mucous membrane at the introitus.

hymenal ring: ridge area encircling the hymen; the dividing line between the vagina and vestibule.

hyperventilation: rate of respiration higher than that required to maintain normal partial pressure of carbon dioxide in the blood, often accompanied by dizziness, chest pain, and tingling of the extremities.

hypothalamus: portion of the diencephalon, lying beneath the thalamus and forming the floor and part of the wall of the third ventricle, joined with the pituitary gland below; most important group of endocrine gland in the body; regulates body growth, development, metabolism, and homeostasis; controls hunger, sex, sleep, and thirst centers; controls hormone production in the glands of the body; controls the autonomic nervous system.

integumentary system: skin (and its derivatives, like hair and nails); provides the external protective covering of the body.

interstitial cells (Leydig cells): cells located in the loose connective tissues surrounding the seminiferous tubules that produce androgen (most importantly testosterone), which are secreted into the surrounding interstitial fluid.

introitus: general term for the entrance to a cavity or space, such as the vagina (introitus, vaginae).

labia: lips; (singular is labium).

labia majora: the greater lip of the pudendum: an elongated fold running downward and backward from the mons pubis.

labia minora: lesser lip of the pudendum: a small fold of skin located between the labium majus and the vaginal introitus; inner lip.

lactic acid: end product of glycolysis, which provides energy anaerobically in skeletal muscle during heavy exercise.

lactobacillus: bacteria in the human mouth, vagina, and intestinal tract; produces lactic acid.

leukocyte: white blood cell.

libido: sex drive or appetite.

ligament: band of regular fibrous tissue that connects bones.

liver: large gland in the right upper abdomen that stores and filters blood, secretes bile, and coverts sugar into glycogen, which it stores.

lumbar: region of the back and side between the ribs and pelvis.

luteinizing hormone (LH): hormone secreted by the anterior pituitary that stimulates ovulation; stimulates progesterone secretion by the corpus luteum in the ovary, and readies the mammary glands for milk secretion in females; stimulates the interstitial cells of the testis to produce testosterone in males.

macrophage: white blood cell (mononuclear phagocyte) present in a number of tissues that engulfs bacteria and foreign debris; may be fixed or wandering; arises from stem cells in the bone marrow.

maculopapular rash: both macular and popular, as an eruption consisting of both macules and papules; a.k.a., goose flesh, goose pimples, or goose bumps.

medial: nearer the midline of the body.

meiosis: special method of cell division, occurring in maturation of the sex cells, by means of which each daughter nucleus receives half the number of chromosomes as the parent cell (see also spermatogenesis).

menopause: termination of ovulation and menstruation, which may be caused by the hypothalamus.

mitosis: method of indirect division of all cells (except sex cells) consisting of a complex of various processes, in which the two daughter nuclei receive identical complements of the number of chromosomes characteristic of the somatic cells of the species.

motor neurons: neurons that conduct impulses from the brain towards the spinal cord or out of the brain and spinal cord into cranial or spinal nerves to effectors that may be either muscles or glands; a.k.a., efferent neurons.

motor nerve: nerve that carries impulses leaving the brain and spinal cord, and destined for effectors.

mucosa: mucous membrane.

mucous membrane: membrane lining a body cavity that opens to the exterior (digestive, respiratory, urinary, and reproductive tracts).

mucus: sticky, thick fluid secretion of goblet cells, mucous cells from mucous glands and mucous membranes, that may moisturize, protect, and lubricate.

muscle, adductor, great: (adductor magnus) situated on the inside thigh; deep part adducts (draws together) high and superficial part extends.

muscle bulbocavernosus: see muscle, bulbospongiosus and muscle, sphincter vaginae.

muscle bulbospongiosus: in the male: contracts the bulbous urethra of the penis to empty urine during urination and semen during ejaculation; in the female: contracts the clitoral bulbs narrowing the vaginal introitus; during orgasm, contracts the clitoral bulbs and vagina; see muscle, bulbocavernosus and muscle, sphincter vaginae.

muscle, compressor urethrae: inner ring-like band of muscle surrounding the urethra and vagina; action: compresses with muscle, sphincter urethrovaginalis.

muscle, compressor vaginae: the muscle, bulbospongiosus in the female.

muscle, gluteal, great: (gluteus maximus) large muscles in the buttocks, which extend, adduct, and rotate the thigh laterally.

muscle, ischiocavernosus: insertion: crus penis and crus clitoridis; action: maintains erection of penis and clitoris.

muscle, levator ani: name applied collectively to important muscular components of the pelvic diaphragm, including the muscles, pubococcygeus (levator prostatae and pubovaginalis), the puborectalis, and the iliococcygeus.

muscle, pubococcygesus: pubococcygeal muscle: a name applied to the anterior (dominant) portion of the levator ani group of perineal muscles, action: helps support pelvic viscera, resists increases in intraabdominal pressure, and may assist in the control of the urinary bladder; PC muscle.

muscle, puborectalis: puborectal muscle: name applied to a portion of the levator ani having a more lateral origin from the pubic bone and continuous posteriorly with the corresponding muscle of the opposite side (sling muscle around the vagina and rectum).

muscle, pubovaginalis: pubovaginal muscle: name applied to a part of the anterior portion of the pubococcygeus muscle, which is inserted into the urethra and vagina (mid-muscle of the vagina).

muscle, rectovesicalis: rectovesical muscle: band of fibers connecting the longitudinal musculature of the rectum with the external coat of the bladder.

muscle, smooth: tissue specialized for contraction, composed of smooth muscle fibers (cells), located in the walls of hollow internal organs and innervated by autonomic motor neurons.

muscle, sphincter urethrae: sphincter muscle of the urethra, action: ring-like band that compresses the membranous part of the urethra.

muscle, sphincter urethrovaginalis: most anterior of two ring-like bands of muscles around the female urethra and vagina; with compressor urethrae (muscle, sphincter urethrae).

muscle, sphincter vaginae: superficial perineal fascia and pouch are split into right and left parts and contain the bulbospongiosus, which is split into right and left parts. The "split" muscles called the bulbospongiosus form the sphincter vaginae. See also muscle, bulbocavernosus and bulbospongiosus.

muscle tissue: tissue specialized to produce motion in response to muscle action potentials by its qualities of contractility, extensibility, elasticity, and excitability; types include skeletal, cardiac, and smooth.

myotonia: distortion or impairment of voluntary movement, as in a spasm (dystonia), involving increased muscular irritability and contractility with decreased power of relaxation.

negative feedback: principle governing most control systems; a mechanism of response in which a stimulus initiates actions that reverse or reduce the stimulus.

nerve: cable-like bundle of neurons (nerve cells) that replays nerve impulses between the body and central nervous system.

nerve impulse: wave of depolarization and repolarization that self-propagates along the plasma membrane of a neuron; also called a nerve action potential.

nervous system: fast-acting control system that triggers muscle contraction or gland secretion.

neuron: one of the billions of interconnected nerve cells that carry electrical signals at high speed and make up the nervous system (brain, spinal cord, and nerves).

neurotransmitter: any of a group of substances released on excitation from a nerve cell that produces an action on another cell.

nipple: pigmented, wrinkled projection on the surface of the breast; location of the openings of the lactiferous ducts for milk release.

nocturnal tumescence: penile or clitoral erections during rapid eye movement (REM) sleep phases.

nucleus: control center of a cell; contains chromosomes.

oogonia: primordial female germ cells that develop into primary oocytes in the fetal ovary.

opioids: any of a group of naturally occurring peptides that bind at or otherwise influence opiate receptors of cell membranes; they may have either opiate-like or opiate antagonist effects; include the dynorphins, endorphins, and enkephalins.

organ: part of the body formed of two or more different kinds of tissues with a special function and usually recognizable shape.

orgasm: acme, apex, or period of greatest intensity, as in sexual excitement; a.k.a., climax.

orgasmic reflex: term (used only in this text) for the involuntary reflexive contractions of the bulbospongiosus muscles of the clitoral bulbs during the female orgasm (may also be known as urethrovaginal reflex or female "ejaculation").

ovarian cycle: sequence of changes, repeated about every 28 days that causes follicle development, ovulation, and corpus luteum formation in the ovary.

ovary: female gonad that produces oocytes and the estrogens, progesterone, inhibin and relaxin hormones.

ovulation: rupture of a mature ovarian follicle into the pelvic cavity.

ovum: female reproductive or germ cell; egg cell.

oxygen: gas found in the air that enters the bloodstream through the lungs and needed by body cells to release energy from glucose.

oxytocin: hormone secreted by the neurosecretory cells in the paraventricular and supraoptic nuclei of the hypothalamus that stimulates contraction of smooth muscle in the pregnant uterus and myoepithelial cells around the ducts of mammary glands.

parasympathetic nervous system: a subdivision of the ANS, having cell bodies of preganglionic neurons in nuclei in the brain stem and in the lateral gray horn of the sacral portion of the spinal cord; primarily concerned with activities that conserve and restore body energy; parasympathetic neurons may cause clitoral and penile erections and may also play a role during orgasm.

pars intermedia: narrow band of erectile tissue extending from the commissura bulborum to the glans of the clitoris.

pelvic diaphragm: separating membrane of the pelvic bone.

pelvic splanchnic nerves: consist of preganglionic parasympathetic axons from the levels of S2, S3, and S4 that supply the urinary bladder, reproductive organs, the sigmoid colon, and rectum.

pelvis: basin-shaped bony structure composed of the pelvic girdle, sacrum, and coccyx.

penis: male organ of copulation and urination; used to deposit semen into the female vagina..

perineum: pelvic floor; space between the anus to the scrotum in males and to the vulva in females.

peripheral nervous system (PNS): part of the nervous system; lies outside the central nervous system, consisting of nerves and ganglia.

permeability: property of membranes that permits passage of molecules and ions.

pH: measure of the concentration of hydrogen ions in a solution; the scale extends from 0 to 14, with a value of seven expressing neutrality, value lower than seven expressing increasing acidity, and values higher than seven expressing alkalinity.

phagocyte: name for white blood cells, including neutrophils and macrophages that engulf and digest disease-causing microorganisms.

pheromone: any biochemical substance produced by one individual that changes the behavior of another person.

pituitary gland: neuroendocrine gland attached under the hypothalamus that serves to regulate the gonads, thyroid, adrenal cortex, lactation, and water balance.

positive feedback: feedback that tends to cause the level of a variable to change in the same direction as an initial change.

posterior: back of an organism, organ, or part; the dorsal surface (opposed to *anterior*).

premature ejaculation: before the intended time or rapid.

prepuce: highly flexible fold of skin covering the head (glans) of the clitoris or penis.

primary follicle (preantral follicle): immature oocyte covered by multiple layers of granulosa cells but without antrum.

primary oocytes: female germ cell in the diplotene stage of first meiotic division.

primordial follicle: immature oocyte covered by a single layer of granulosa cells.

progesterone: principal progestational hormone of the body, liberated by the corpus luteum, placenta, and in minute amounts by the adrenal cortex; prepares the uterus for implantation of a fertilized ovum and the mammary glands for milk secretion.

psychogenic erection: erection triggered by the higher cerebral centers and hypothalamus; mental or psychic erection.

psychovasoneuromuscular event: an event which involves the psyche or brain, vascular or blood flow, neurons, and muscles.

puberty: time of life during which the secondary sex characteristics begin to appear and the capability for sexual reproduction is possible; usually occurs between the ages of 10 and 17.

receptor: specialized cell or a distal portion of a neuron that responds to a specific sensory stimulus, such as touch, pressure, cold, light, or sound, and converts it to an electrical signal.

reflex: fast response to a change (stimulus) in the internal or external environment that attempts to restore homeostasis.

reflexogenic erection: erection initiated by a reflex.

refractory period: a time period during which an excitable cell (neuron or muscle fiber) cannot respond to a stimulus that is usually adequate to evoke an action potential.

sacrum: triangular bone just below the lumbar formed by five fused vertebrae (sacral vertebrae) and above the tail bone.

secondary sex characteristic: characteristic that develops at puberty under the influence of sex hormones but is not directly involved in sexual reproduction; examples are distribution of body hair, voice pitch, body shape, bone growth, and muscle development.

secretion: production and release from a cell or a gland of a physiologically active substance.

semen: fluid discharged at ejaculation by a male that consists of a mixture of sperm and the secretions of the seminiferous tubules, seminal vesicles, prostate, and bulbourethral (Cowper's) glands.

seminal vesicle (vesicula seminalis): either of the paired pouches attached to the posterior part of the urinary bladder; the duct of each joins the ductus deferens to form the ejaculatory duct.

seminiferous tubules: highly convoluted tubes within the testes that form spermatozoa or sperm.

sensation: state of awareness of internal or external body conditions.

sensory nerve: nerve that contains processes of sensory neurons and carries nerve impulses to the central nervous system.

sensory neuron: neuron that carry sensory information from cranial and spinal nerves into the brain and spinal cord or from a lower to a higher level in the spinal cord and brain; a.k.a., afferent neurons.

sensory receptor: dendritic end organs, or parts of other cell types, specialized to respond to a stimulus.

sex chromosomes: the 23rd pair of chromosomes, designated X and Y; determines individual's genetic sex (XX = female; XY = male).

sinusoid: large, thin-walled, leaky type of capillary having large intercellular clefts that may allow proteins and blood cells to pass from a tissue into the bloodstream; present in the liver, anterior pituitary, parathyroid glands, red bone marrow, clitoris, and penis.

somatic nerves: portion of peripheral nervous system consisting of somatic sensory (afferent) neurons and somatic motor (efferent) neurons.

somatic nervous system: portion of the peripheral nervous system consisting of somatic sensory (afferent) neurons and somatic motor (efferent) neurons; may play a role during ejaculation.

sperm: mature male germ cell; a.k.a., spermatozoon; plural spermatozoa.

spermatocyte: parent cell of a spermatid.

spermatogenesis: formation and development of sperm (male gamete) in the seminiferous tubules of the testes; takes about 74 days to complete the maturation.

spermiogenesis: the maturation of spermatids into sperm.

spermatogonium: plural spermatogonia, the undifferentiated male germ cell, originating in the seminiferous tubule and dividing into two primary spermatocytes.

sphincter: circular muscle, constricts an opening (see muscle).

spinal cord: mass of nervous tissue located in the vertebral canal from which 31 pairs of spinal nerves originate; provides a conduction pathway to and from the brain and is so thin it only weighs an ounce, less than 4 percent of the brain itself.

spinal nerve: one of the 31 pairs of nerves that originate on the spinal cord from posterior and anterior roots.

SRY gene: sex-determining region on the Y short arm of the chromosome, this gene makes an enzyme or protein (testis-determining factor) that is necessary for testes to develop.

steroid: one of a group of lipids that include cholesterol, certain hormones, and vitamins.

stimulus: any stress that changes a controlled condition; any change in the internal or external environment that excites a sensory receptor, a neuron or a muscle fiber; plural stimuli.

sympathetic nervous system (SNS): subdivision of the ANS, having cell bodies of preganglionic neurons in the lateral gray columns of the thoracic segment and the first two lumbar segments of the spinal cord; primarily concerned with processes involving the expenditure of energy; the fight, fright, and flight subdivision; regulated by the hypothalamus and may cause emission of semen, ejaculation and detumescence of erections.

symphysis pubis: joint formed by the union of the bodies of the pubic bones in the median plane by a thick mass of fibrocartilage.

testis: male primary sex organ that produces sperm; male gonad; testicle; plural testes.

testosterone: androgenic hormone produced by the interstitial (Leydig) cells of the testis in response to the luteinizing hormone (LH) of the anterior pituitary and regulated by the hypothalamus; needed for sperm development; together with a second androgen (dihydrotestosterone or DHT) controls the development of male reproductive organs, secondary sex characteristics, and body growth.

thermoreceptor: sensory receptor; detects changes in temperature.

thirst center: cluster of neurons in the hypothalamus sensitive to the osmotic pressure of extra cellular fluid; produces sensation of thirst.

transudation: passage of serum or other body fluid through a blood vessel as a result of hydrodynamic forces.

tunica albuginea: a dense, white, fibrous sheath enclosing a part or organ such as the penis.

urethra: duct from the urinary bladder to the exterior that conveys urine in females, and urine and semen in males.

urethral ridge: fibrous interior of the anterior vaginal wall that shields and contains the fused urethra.

urogenital diaphragm: separating membrane within the pelvic bone; essentially keeps the internal organs from falling out of the body.

uterine tube: duct that transports ova from the ovary to the uterus; fallopian tube or oviduct.

uterus: hollow, muscular organ in females that is the site of menstruation, implantation, development of the fetus, and labor.

vagina: fibromuscular sheath from the cervix to the vestibule; receives the penis during coitus; serves as newborn's birth canal.

vasoconstriction: decrease in the size of the lumen of a blood vessel caused by constriction of the smooth muscles in the wall of the vessel.

vasodilation: relaxation of the walls of the blood vessel that increases or widens the vessel, and maintains or lowers blood pressure.

vein: conveys blood from tissues to the heart.

vellus: fine body hair.

vestibule: small space or cavity at the beginning of a canal, especially the inner ear, larynx, mouth, nose, and vagina.

vulva: collective designation for the external genitalia of the female.

white matter: bundles of myelinated and unmyelinated axons located in the brain and spinal cord.

INDEX

Leukocytes, 15
Libido (see also sex drive): 25, female, 34, male, 28-29, 34
Lips, 25, 34, 37-39
Love, 1, 31, 35, 38-39, 67

Macrophages, 15
Maculopapular rash (sex flush), 41, 49, 60
Marriage, 31, 35, 67
Medication, 31
Menopause, 34-35
Menstrual cycle, 15, 34
Metabolic rate, 19
Microbes, 15
Mitosis, 32
Mons pubis, 9, 41
Morphine, 68
Mouth, 39
Mucous glands, 10, 13
Mucous membrane, 14
Mucus, 14, 45
Muscle, bulbospongiosus:
    female, 3, 16, 25, 47, 57, 59-61
    male, 3, 24, 62
Muscle, clitoral bulb, (see muscles, bulbospongiosus)
Muscle, compressor urethrae, 11, 15, 25
Muscle, vaginae, (see bulbospongiosus, female)
Muscle, gluteus, great (maximus):
    female, 54; male, 49, 60
Muscle, ischiocavernosus:
    female, 3, 50, 59; male, 3, 62
Muscle, levator ani: female, 12, 25, 43, 48, 53-56; male, 56-57
Muscle, medial adductor, great (adductor magnus),
Muscle, pelvic floor: female, 25, 57, 60-61; male, 60-61
Muscle, pubococcygeus (PC):
    female, 16, 25, 48, 52, 56-57, 59, 61; male, 62
Muscle, puborectalis, 16, 25, 56, 59
Muscle, pubovaginalis, 16, 25, 56, 59
Muscle, rectovesicalis, 15, 25, 56, 59
Muscle, smooth: female, 12; male, 5
Muscle, sphincter, anal: female, 25, 57, 59; male, 24. 62
Muscle, sphincter, urethra (internal and external), female, 11
Muscle, sphincter, urethrovaginalis, 11, 15, 25, 56, 59
Myotonia, 51, 53

ABOUT THE AUTHOR

Royal Yu and his wife were married in 1959 and reside in the Aloha State of Hawaii with their four children and spouses, and seven grandchildren.

Yu began writing this book as a legacy for his children. During his intensive research, however, he decided to share some of the "Secrets."

Royal hopes that his book about "the birds and the bees" will enhance your marriage.

Like great sex, an author always needs positive feedback! Contact him at:

royalyu@royalpublishingllc.com

Mahalo (thank you) and A-L-O-H-A!

Royal Yu